MANAGING
DYSFUNCTIO..

Michael Cummings MD FRCP
Consultant Physician and Honorary Reader,
Diabetes and Endocrinology,
Academic Department of Diabetes and Endocrinology,
Queen Alexandra Hospital,
Southwick Hill Road, Cosham,
Portsmouth, Hampshire

ALTMAN

Published by Altman Publishing, 7 Ash Copse, Bricket Wood, St Albans, Herts, AL2 3YA, England

First published 2006

Typeset in 10/12 Optima by Scribe Design Ltd, Ashford, Kent
Printed in Great Britain by Ingersoll Printers Ltd, Wembley

ISBN 1 86036 032 7

A catalogue record for this book is available from the British Library

∞ Printed on acid-free text paper, manufactured in accordance with ANSI/NISO Z39.48-1992 (Permanence of Paper)

CONTENTS

Preface   iv

1 Why treat erectile dysfunction?   1

2 How are penile erections achieved?   7

3 What causes erectile dysfunction?   15

4 How do I assess the patient with erectile
   dysfunction in my surgery?   23

5 What practical issues should I consider
   before offering treatment?   35

6 Management algorithm   41

7 Oral therapy: when and how?   43

8 Invasive pharmacological therapy:
   when and how?   51

9 Are there any alternative approaches
   to drug therapy?   59

10 Special considerations   67

11 What additional support is available
   for myself and my patients?   77

Index   79

PREFACE

At medical school, I do not recall being taught about erectile dysfunction (ED). This condition, however, is extremely common and thought to affect 1 in 20 men within the UK and up to 1 in 4 transiently. It is essential therefore that health care professionals have at least a basic understanding of the condition. It is inevitable that more and more patients will seek your advice for this complaint within a variety of settings, both in primary and specialist care. Since the introduction of phosphodiesterase type 5 inhibitors, the first class of effective oral agents for ED, this has meant a greater shift of emphasis than ever towards the management of ED within primary care.

This book aims to provide a concise account of the management of ED aimed at health care professionals within primary care, such as general practitioners and practice nurses. Whilst providing sufficient background to understand the nature of ED and how to assess and manage the condition, it does not dwell on detailed academia. In particular, it focuses upon the practical issues of management, incorporating an algorithmic approach to treating ED. Each chapter concludes with key learning points and provides further relevant sources of more detailed information if required.

In the twenty-first century, we have effective options to treat ED, the hindrance is often knowing how and when to use them.

MHC

1 WHY TREAT ERECTILE DYSFUNCTION?

Traditionally for health care professionals (HCPs) and patients, erectile dysfunction (ED) has never been a comfortable area to discuss for many reasons. In consequence, there have been many barriers (see Table 1.1) that have led to the patient and his partner receiving inadequate advice and treatment, with sometimes devastating consequences. The burden of this disorder is now recognised as substantive given the frequency with which it is observed (see Figure 1.1). It is thought that 5% of the UK male population have permanent ED whilst a further 15% suffer with ED intermittently.

Traditional barriers to treatment

Discussing sexual dysfunction is perceived as more difficult for the patient and the HCP compared with other health care issues and has

Table 1.1 Barriers to treating ED

ED – a taboo subject
ED – not a serious disorder
Poor understanding of the aetiology of ED
Lack of effective treatment
Lack of health care professionals with an interest in ED
Economic considerations

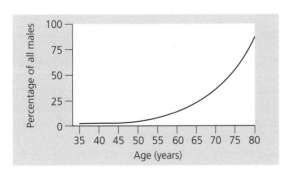

Figure 1.1 The prevalence of ED in the general population.

often been considered a taboo subject. For the patient, the primary issue is typically around embarrassment and the feeling of inadequacy, coupled with a poor understanding of the problem associated with misconceptions. For the HCP, a number of complex issues have contributed. Should ED be prioritised for treatment in a state health system compared with other much more serious conditions? After all, nobody has ever died of ED and for many patients, the problem develops in later life when egg fertilisation is no longer a relevant factor. Whilst some HCPs have recognised the impact ED is having upon an individual, they have been unaware of effective treatment or specialist centres that can offer treatment. Treating ED can also be expensive and time consuming.

Fortunately, the last decade has seen a considerable advance in our understanding of ED, leading to removal of many of the original barriers. Robust scales have been developed and validated that can reliably assess the presence and severity of ED as well as any impact upon quality of life. With knowledge of the biochemical mechanisms that contribute to the development of ED it has been possible to develop effective pharmacological approaches to the treatment of this condition. In particular, the introduction of oral phosphodiesterase type 5 (PDE5) inhibitors has captured the imagination of the national and international press, which in turn has led to raised public awareness and greater knowledge and demand for treatment. It is now recognised that ED is a common, eminently treatable disorder that should not be ignored! In consequence, many HCPs in primary care feel able to offer assessment and first-line treatment options with back-up for more invasive or complex treatment strategies being provided by specialist centres. These include urologists, diabetologists, psychosexual counsellors, specialist GPs and nurses, and others.

The psychological benefits of treating ED

The presence of ED has now been shown to be unequivocally associated with significant impairment in quality of life, affecting both psychological and social aspects of the patient's well-being. ED can lead to performance anxiety, resulting in generalised anxiety and depression, and marital strain is not uncommon. For some groups of patients this can be very demoralising, leading to other perils. For instance, in diabetic males, depression can result in lack of motivation, which has a negative impact upon glycaemic control and management of other vascular risk factors. Importantly, a number of studies have also demonstrated that treating ED can improve quality of life.

How does improving quality of life compare with treating serious physical disorders such as cancers and ischaemic heart disease? This question, embracing the concept of quantity versus quality of life, has vexed philosophers and will continue to do so for many years to come. Nevertheless, we already *are* treating many disorders that affect quality but not quantity of life. Examples include mental disorders, benign prostate disorders, and many skin disorders, to name a few. Moreover, national bodies such as NICE (the National Institute for Clinical Excellence) recognise and incorporate assessment upon quality of life (QOL) within their guidance. The National Service Framework for Diabetes states that 'regular surveillance and effective management...of ED can reduce the impact...on the QOL of people with diabetes'.

The physical benefits of treating ED

Chapter 5 highlights the importance of a cardiovascular assessment in patients with ED. Healthy sexual function can be a good form of exercise associated with its inherent benefits. However, ED is often associated with underlying cardiovascular disease and has been identified by some as an independent risk factor for vascular disorders. Thus, taking ED seriously with an appropriate assessment may lead to the discovery of other hitherto unrecognised cardiac disease, leading to earlier treatment. Moreover, it is recognised that a high percentage of patients with ED (up to 40%) may have underlying diabetes, a significant number being 'new' cases. Successful treatment is often associated with improved motivation and attitude to other co-morbid conditions.

Economic considerations of treating ED

Prior to the development of oral PDE5 inhibitors, it was often perceived that relatively little cost was attached to the management of ED nationally. The introduction and unlimited use of PDE5 inhibitors was thought to have been unaffordable, which led to the Department of Health issuing guidelines on the use of treatments of ED, limiting the patients groups that were eligible for treatment and the number of treatments per week that were prescribable within the state health system (see

Table 1.2 Costs incurred in primary and secondary care for ED pre-(1998–99) and post- (1999–2000) launch of sildenafil within the Portsmouth district, UK

	1998–1999 (pre-sildenafil)	1999–2000 (post-sildenafil)
Secondary care out-patient attendances	£100 538	£26 231
Secondary care prescribing	£16 391	£4064
Primary care prescribing	£94 262	£183 093
Penile implants	£8000	£7600
Total	£219 191	£220 988

Chapter 5). Since their introduction, it has been shown that in a typical health district, there has been an uplift in the number of men being treated for ED with the total costs for management remaining similar (see Table 1.2). Increases in drug budgets by primary care physicians were offset by a similar decrease in the costs associated with specialist care and assessment and the use of more complex treatment regimens.

Key points

- Traditionally ED has been a taboo subject with ineffective treatment strategies and few HCPs offering advice and management.
- The psychological and physical benefits of treating ED are now compelling.
- A greater understanding of the mechanisms leading to ED has led to the development of effective treatment strategies (in particular PDE5 inhibitors) for this condition.
- The treatment of ED within the state health system remains affordable.
- The majority of men with ED can be successfully treated.

Further reading

Ashton-Key M, Sadler M, Walmsley B, Holmes S, Randall S, Cummings MH. (2002) UK department of health guidance on prescribing for impotence following the introduction of sildenafil: potential to contain costs in the average health authority district. *Pharmacoeconomics* **20**(12), 839–46.

Cummings MH, Meeking D, Warburton F, Alexander WD. (1997) The diabetic male's perception of erectile dysfunction. *Practical Diabetes International* **14**(4), 100–12.

De Beradis G, Franciosi M, Belfiglio M. (2002) Erectile dysfunction and quality of life in type 2 diabetic patients. *Diabetes Care* **25**, 284–91.

Department of Health (2001) National Service Framework for Diabetes (http://www.publications.doh.gov.uk/nsf/diabetes/)

Gazzaruso C, Giordanetti S, De Amici E, Bertone G, Falcone C, Geroldi D, Fratino C, Solerte S, Garzaniti A. (2004) Relationship between erectile dysfunction and silent myocardial ischaemia in apparently uncomplicated type 2 diabetic patients. *Circulation* **110**, 226.

NIH (1993) National Institutes of Health Consensus Development Panel on Impotence. *Journal of the American Medical Association* **270**, 83–90.

2 HOW ARE PENILE ERECTIONS ACHIEVED?

In order to understand the pathophysiology of ED, it is important to recognise the normal processes by which an erection is obtained. Thirty years ago, it was conceived by many HCPs that ED was a 'condition of the mind', implying that most cases were psychological in origin. Subsequent studies confirmed the role of testosterone in determining libido and sexual function, leading to the trend of attempting to improve tumescence with administration of this hormone in most cases of ED regardless of potential cause. In the 1990s, the role of nitric oxide in facilitating adequate blood flow and penile smooth muscle relaxation was discovered, hailing the development of a potential cure for the condition. It is now recognised, however, that the development of a physiological erection is complex, requiring the sophisticated co-ordination of multiple organs to achieve tumescence. In addition, at the cellular level, there is a complex interaction of multiple chemical messengers that determine penile smooth muscle tone. Thus, it is perhaps not surprising that there is no one approach to treatment that will achieve success in all patients with ED.

In considering the approaches to treating ED, it is best to consider the physiology of achieving tumescence at three levels:

- the multiple organ co-ordinated response to achieve erections
- the physiological mechanisms leading to erection within the penis itself
- the biochemical pathways leading to relaxation of the penile smooth muscle cell.

The multiple organ co-ordinated response to achieve erections

Figure 2.1 shows the various organs that activate the penile tissue response, ultimately leading to an erection. The initiating event is enhanced libido and it is thought that this response to external signals is mediated through the hypothalamus. Signals from the hypothalamus

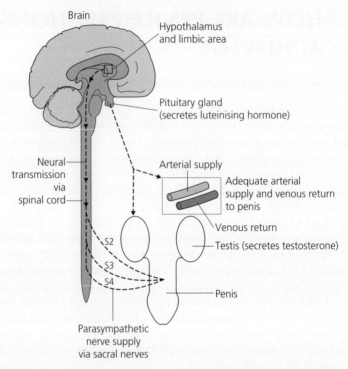

Figure 2.1 The multi-organ response required to achieve tumescence.

are then transmitted along the descending tracts of the spinal cord supplying the spinal nuclei which innervate the penis. Knowledge of the chemical messengers within the hypothalamus have been exploited to promote the development of drug therapy to treat ED (see Chapter 7). These include dopamine (in particular D2 receptor agonists), alpha-adrenergic receptor agonists and 5-hydroxytryptamine.

Adequate supply of testosterone is central to increased libido, which is dependent upon an intact gonadal axis involving biofeedback between the hypothalamus, pituitary gland and testes (see Figure 2.2). Evidence suggests that testosterone acts upon the hypothalamus, promoting an enhanced dopaminergic response, and may also affect the availability or action of nitric oxide within the penile smooth muscle itself. Alterations in the hormonal milieu that affect the testosterone axis,

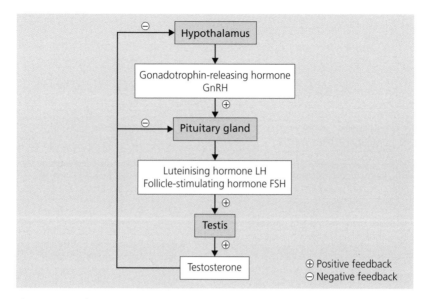

Figure 2.2 The testosterone axis.

such as abnormalities in prolactin and thyroid metabolism, may also adversely affect erectile function.

The physiological mechanisms leading to erection within the penis itself

Enhanced libido and the higher centres' neural response leads to stimulation of the parasympathetic nervous system via the nerve roots S2, S3 and S4 (see Figure 2.3). This results in vasodilation of the penile artery (a branch of the internal pudendal artery) and its tributary vessels, in particular the helicine arteries that supply the sinusoidal spaces within the trabecular smooth muscle of the penis. Increased blood supply to the penis, perhaps ten times the basal flow, is coupled with penile smooth muscle relaxation, facilitating accumulation of blood within the sinusoidal spaces. As penile erection develops with the accumulation of pooled blood, there is compression of the venous plexi situated within the periphery of the penis, thereby inhibiting venous return. Sympathetic nerve stimulation (originating in the nerve roots T11–L2)

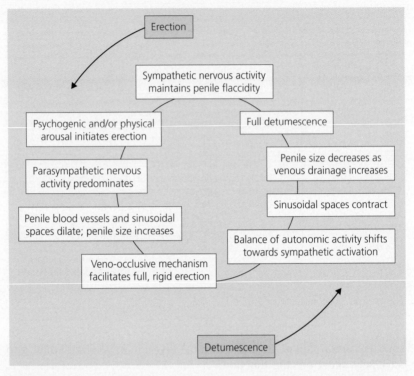

Figure 2.3 The mechanism of penile erection. Adapted from Cummings MH, Alexander WD. (1999) Erectile dysfunction in patients with diabetes. *Hospital Medicine* **60**, 638–44.

results in orgasm. Stimulation of the sympathetic nervous system is also responsible for initiating detumescence with a reversal of the above process.

The biochemical pathways leading to relaxation of the penile smooth muscle cell

Knowledge of the biochemical mediators involved in the process of smooth muscle relaxation has perhaps been the greatest breakthrough in the development of treatment strategies for ED. The final common

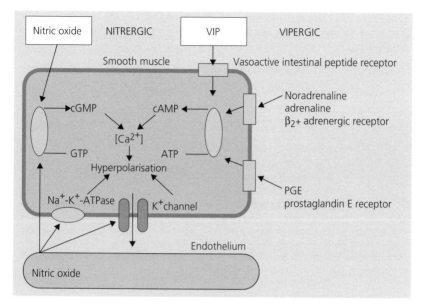

Figure 2.4 The biochemical pathways leading to penile smooth muscle relaxation. Adapted with permission from Christ GJ. (1995) The penis as a vascular organ. The importance of corporal smooth muscle tone in the control of erection. *Urology Clinics of North America* **22**, 727–45.

pathway leading to smooth muscle relaxation is the decrease in available intracellular calcium (see Figure 2.4). This is achieved by augmentation of the intracellular messengers, cyclic AMP and cyclic GMP. In turn the intracellular concentration of cyclic AMP and GMP is dependent upon the availability of stimuli that promote their production and release as well as metabolism. Often, this involves stimulation of a receptor situated on the smooth muscle wall, such as nitric oxide, prostaglandin E1 or vasoactive intestinal polypeptide (VIP) (see Table 2.1). Conversely, there are chemical stimuli that promote the reverse process of smooth muscle constriction and it is the relative balance between the availability of multiple chemical substances, in part under the auspices of the autonomic nervous system, that determine the penile smooth muscle response.

Table 2.1 Biochemical mediators of penile smooth muscle tone*

	Contractile	Relaxant
Neuronal	**Noradrenaline** Neuropeptide Y (NPY)	**Nitric oxide** **Acetylcholine** **Vasoactive intestinal** **polypeptide (VIP)** Calcitonin gene related peptide (CGRP)
Circulating	Arginine vasopressin	
Local	**Endothelin-1** Thromboxane A_2 Prostaglandin $F_{2\alpha}$ Prostaglandin I_2 Angiotensin II	**Nitric oxide** Prostaglandin A_2 Prostaglandin I_2 Histamine Adenosine triphosphate

*From Eardley I, Sethia K. (eds) (1998) *Erectile Dysfunction: Current Investigation and Management*, pp. 1–19. London: Mosby-Wolfe.

Key points

- Achieving erections requires a complex interaction between the central, peripheral and autonomic nervous systems, the endocrine system, adequate penile blood flow and the penile tissue.
- The critical responses within the penis are dilation of the penile artery and its tributaries (in particular the helicine arteries) as well as smooth muscle relaxation facilitating accumulation of blood within the sinusoidal spaces.
- Smooth muscle tone within the penis is determined by the relative interactions of chemical substances that promote relaxation and constriction, chiefly acting through their chemical messengers cyclic AMP and GMP, which ultimately determine the availability of intracellular calcium.

Further reading

Eardley I, Sethia K. (1998) Anatomy and physiology of erection. In: *Erectile Dysfunction: Current Investigation and Management*. London: Mosby-Wolfe.

Christ GJ. (1995) The penis as a vascular organ. The importance of corporal smooth muscle tone in the control of erection. *Urological Clinics of North America* **22**, 727–45.

Lue TF, Takamura T, Schmidt RA, Palubishos AJ, Tanagho EA. (1983) Hemodynamics of erection in the monkey. *Journal of Urology* **128**, 1237–41.

Saenz de Tejada I, Moreland M. (1993) Physiology of erection, pathophysiology of impotence, and implications of PGE1 in the control of collagen synthesis in the corpus cavernosum. In: Goldstein I, Lue TF (eds), *The Role of Alprostadil in the Diagnosis and Treatment of Erectile Dysfunction*. Princeton: Excerpta Medica.

Further reading

3   WHAT CAUSES ERECTILE DYSFUNCTION?

The physiology of tumescence described in Chapter 2 provides a rationale for the development of ED in most cases. It is recognised, however, that in many cases of ED there can be a causative interplay between multiple factors, both physical and psychological. For instance, it is very common for men to develop perfomance anxiety, thereby further adversely affecting penile responses in men with an underlying physical cause for their ED. Figure 3.1 attempts to show the common conditions associated with ED, whilst Table 3.1 highlights the processes that may be disturbed and thereby implicated in its development.

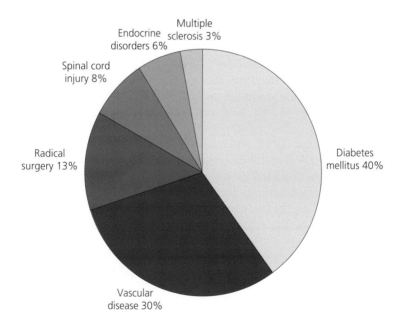

Figure 3.1   Conditions associated with the development of ED. Adapted with permission from Zonszein J. (1995) Diagnosis and management of endocrine disorders of erectile dysfunction. *Urological Clinics of North America* **22**(4), 789–802.

Table 3.1 Factors that may be associated with the development of ED

Neural factors (abnormalities of the parasympathetic nervous system)
Vascular factors (atherosclerosis and endothelial dysfunction)
Functional and structural changes within the corpus cavernosum (primary or
  secondary)
Primary penile abnormalities (for example Peyronie's disease)
Endocrine factors (diabetes mellitus, hypogonadism or thyroid disease)
Iatrogenic factors (drugs, radiotherapy or surgery)
Psychological factors and psychiatric disorders
Venous leaks
Infections (balanitis)
Chronic illnesses (for example malignancy or renal failure)

Neural factors

Many diseases affecting the central, peripheral (autonomic nervous system) have the potential to cause ED.

The most common cause of an autonomic neuropathy is diabetes mellitus (see Chapter 10) but other causes include alcohol-related damage, vitamin B12 deficiency, malignancy and amyloidosis. This pathological process interrupts the parasympathetic innervation required for a normal erectile response discussed in Chapter 2.

Diseases of the spinal cord can interfere with normal descending neural impulses. The most common causes include demyelination, trauma and spinal cord compression. It is interesting to note that physiological erections may still be present in spinal cord disorders, due either to the presence of partial or intermittent lesions (for example, multiple sclerosis) or if the lesion is below T12 where the reflex arc remains intact.

Diseases of the central nervous system may affect libido within the arousal centre of the hypothalamus or onward neural transmission. Examples include parkinsonism, demyelination or non-vascular dementia (Alzheimer's disease). Temporal lobe epilepsy may also cause ED, presumably through a mechanism affecting normal function within the hypothalamus.

Vascular factors

Inadequate penile blood flow may occur for two reasons. First, there may be structural lesions, usually atherosclerosis, which restrict blood flow.

Second, despite arteries with apparently normal appearances, there may be an inability of these vessels to vasodilate following innervation by the parasympathetic nervous system (known as endothelial dysfunction). It is probable that the reduced blood flow results in relative ischaemia within the smooth muscle cells, thereby affecting the ability of the corpus cavernosum to relax. Atherosclerotic disease may be generalised, such as that observed in diabetes. Conventional risk factors such as hyperlipidaemia, a premature history of vascular disease, hypertension or smoking increase the risk of endothelial dysfunction or atherosclerosis and therefore the likelihood of ischaemia-induced ED. Alternatively, ED may be due to localised arterial disease, such as narrowings in the external iliac artery (known as 'pelvic steal' syndrome).

Abnormalities of venous drainage are also associated with the development of ED. In some instances, there is a primary abnormality of venous return which prevents the pooling of blood within the sinusoid lakes of the corpus cavernosum. It is now recognised, however, that the majority of cases of so-called venous leakage are the consequence of a problem elsewhere, such as in the smooth muscle itself, or due to distorted anatomy related to penile disorders including Peyronie's disease or previous penile surgery.

Endocrine factors

Diabetes mellitus may affect erectile function in numerous ways and is covered elsewhere (see Chapter 10). Hypogonadism, hyperprolactinaemia and thyroid disorders are also implicated (see Chapter 10). It is widely thought that hypogonadism impedes libido through reduced effect within the hypothalamus, although recent experimental evidence has suggested that the action of nitric oxide, a principal mediator of penile smooth muscle relaxation, may be reduced.

Primary disorders of penile smooth muscle relaxation

Whilst neurovascular disease may precipitate ED though altering the biochemical milieu within the penile smooth muscles that facilitate relaxation, it is clear that some patients may develop impotence through the same ultimate mechanisms although the factors initiating these abnormalities remain obscure.

Table 3.2 Biochemical determinants of smooth muscle tone within the corpus cavernosum that may be affected in ED

	Relaxant	Contractile
Neuronal release	Nitric oxide Acetylcholine Vasoactive intestinal polypeptide	Noradrenaline
Local release	Nitric oxide Vasodilator prostanoids Adenosine triphosphate	Endothelin-1 Vasoconstrictor prostanoids

Considerable research has now identified a number of biochemical mediators that determine penile smooth muscle tone (see Chapter 2). In many cases, it is thought that there is a relative deficiency or excess of factors (or their action) that enhance either relaxation or constriction of these muscle cells. Although disturbances of nitric oxide metabolism or action have been identified as a major contributory factor, several other key factors may be affected (see Table 3.2).

In addition to changes in functionality, the penile structure may be altered. For instance, diabetes is associated with a greater deposition of fibrous tissue in the penile vasculature, corpus cavernosum and nerve fibres that attenuate local vasodilation or smooth muscle relaxation. Whether these changes are the initiating event or a consequence of other mechanisms causing ED is unclear.

Finally, patients may present with primary congenital or acquired disorders of the penis that interrupt the neurovascular supply or the mechanisms of penile smooth muscle relaxation. Examples include Peyronie's disease, penile carcinoma or trauma.

Iatrogenic factors

Drugs

There are now a substantive number of drugs that have been associated with the development of ED (see Table 3.3). For many drugs there is a plausible explanation as to why ED develops. For example, antihypertensive agents may reduce penile perfusion in this susceptible group of patients, many of whom already exhibit evidence of generalised athero-sclerosis. Not all antihypertensive agents appear to be associated with the same risk of precipitating ED (see Table 3.4). Some drugs inhibit the action of circulating testosterone such as spironolactone or cyproterone.

Table 3.3 Drugs associated with the development of ED

Drug type	Comment
Antihypertensive agents	Includes thiazides, beta-blockers, angiotensin-converting enzyme inhibitors, hydralazine, methyldopa, prazosin and clonidine
Antidepressant agents	Tricyclic antidepressants and monoamine oxidase inhibitors
Antipsychotic agents	Phenothiazines (in particular thioridazine and lithium)
Antiarrhythmic agents	Verapamil, flecainide, propafenone, disopyramide
Lipid-lowering agents	Statins, fibrates
Anticonvulsant agents	Carbamazepine, gabapentin
Alcohol	50% likelihood of ED when 40 units or more of alcohol consumed per week
Opiates	
Miscellaneous	Acetazolamide, allopurinol, anabolic steroids, baclofen, bromocriptine, cimetidine, ketoconazole, metoclopramide, non-steroidal anti-inflammatory drugs, oestrogens

Table 3.4 Risks of the development of ED with different classes of antihypertensive agents*

Drug	Difficulty in obtaining erections	Difficulty in maintaining erections
Doxazosin	4.2%	2.8%
Placebo	6.8%	6.8%
Enalapril	8.2%	6.6%
Amlodipine	8.5%	6.8%
Acebutolol	6.9%	8.3%
Chlorthalidone	17.1%	15.7%

*From Grimm RH Jr, Grandits GA, Prineas RJ, McDonald RH, Lewis CE, Flack JM, Yunis C, Svendsen K, Liebson PR, Elmer PJ. (1997) Long-term effects on sexual function of five antihypertensive drugs and nutritional hygienic treatment in hypertensive men and women. Treatment of Mild Hypertension Study (TOMHS) *Hypertension* **29**, 8–14.

Hypnotic agents and major tranquillisers are capable of promoting a hyperprolactinaemic state which inhibits the gonadal axis and release of testosterone. With certain agents, for example lipid lowering agents, it is unclear why ED develops.

Surgery and radiotherapy

Surgery can inadvertently cause ED through a number of mechanisms, principally causing damage to the autonomic nervous system or higher nerve centres, penile blood supply or damage to the penile structure *per se*. One of the most common causes is prostatectomy, whether undertaken transurethrally or retropubically (risk approximately 13.5 and 15.6%, respectively). Other causes include radical cystectomy, anterior or abdominoperineal resection of the rectum or urethroplasty. Penile blood flow may be impaired following aorto-iliac surgery or renal transplant.

Radical radiotherapy to pelvic organ carcinomas (prostate, bladder or rectum) may cause ED, presumably through inducing unwanted neurovascular damage as a result of vasculitic changes.

Psychological factors

Pure psychogenic ED may reflect an underlying psychological disorder such as anxiety or depression and may be related to a life event, or may be endogenous. It is assumed, although not proven, that such disorders affect the arousal mechanisms originating within the hypothalamus. Alternatively, drugs used to treat psychological disorders may be associated with the development of ED *per se* (see above). The same principles apply to patients with underlying psychiatric disorders associated with the development of ED.

It is not uncommon for patients with ED to have concomitant physical and psychological factors precipitating ED, the latter developing in response to the prospect of perceived failure when attempting repeated penetrative intercourse.

Other factors

Any condition associated with penile pain, for example balanitis, may result in ED. In addition, chronic illnesses and malignancy have the potential to promote ED through a variety of mechanisms, both physical and psychological. Finally, chronic renal failure is a notorious precipitant of ED, in particular in patients on dialysis, possibly related to neurovascular factors, penile smooth muscle dysfunction and endocrine factors (hypogonadism and/or hyperprolactinaemia).

Key points

- The aetiology of ED is often multifactorial.
- Neurovascular factors and changes within the penile smooth muscle itself (that affect structure or function) are the principal causes of ED.
- A number of abnormalities affecting the availability or action of biochemical mediators that determine penile smooth muscle tone have been identified.
- Other aetiological factors include endocrine disorders (in particular diabetes and hypogonadism), psychological disorders/psychiatric disease, or iatrogenic factors related to the use of drug therapy, surgery or radiotherapy.
- Most causes of ED are predictable, knowing the normal physiological pathways responsible for achieving tumescence.

Further reading

Aydos K, Baltaci S, Saglam M. (1996) Ultrastuctural changes in corpus cavernosa in vascular erectile dysfunction. *International Urology and Nephrology* **28**, 275–85.

Eardley I, Sethia K. (1998) Pathophysiology of erectile dysfunction. In: *Erectile Dysfunction: Current Investigation and Management*. London: Mosby-Wolfe.

Feldman HA, Goldstein I, Hatzicchritsou DG, Krane RJ, Mckinlay JB. (1994) Impotence and its medical and psychosexual correlates: results of the Massachusetts Male Aging Study. *Journal of Urology* **151**, 54–61.

Johannes CB, Araujo AB, Feldman HA, Derby CA, Kleinman KP, Mckinlay JB. (2000) Incidence of erectile dysfunction in men 40 to 69 years old: longitudinal results from the Massachusetts Male Aging Study. *Journal of Urology* **163**, 460–3.

Zonszein J. (1995) Diagnosis and management of endocrine disorders of erectile dysfunction. *Urological Clinics of North America* **22**(4), 789–802.

4 HOW DO I ASSESS THE PATIENT WITH ERECTILE DYSFUNCTION IN MY SURGERY?

General observations

Discussing ED can be a painful and embarrassing experience for the patient and HCP. It is important that the HCP has a strategy for managing the condition. Too often in the past HCPs have trivialised the problem, often as a result of inadequate knowledge on how to assess or manage the patient, embarrassment or even lack of knowledge of appropriate specialist centres that offer treatment for ED. Responding to the patient that ED is likely to improve spontaneously with time is a myth, whether of organic or psychological origin, yet was often quoted to avoid further discussions of the condition. Thus it may be that the initial approach in the GP surgery is to ascertain the nature of the problem and then ask the patient to return to a less hurried and more appropriate environment so the condition can be more fully assessed and discussed. With the advent of effective oral therapy, it is becoming more commonplace for ED to be managed in the primary care setting either by the GP or practice nurse. Thus it is important for the HCP to be empathic and have an understanding of the relevant points to address in the history and examination. This should lead to a management plan that can be effected either within the HCP's own practice or by a referral route to the most appropriate specialist centre elsewhere.

History

Defining the problem

First, ascertain what the patient means by impotence or erectile dysfunction. Previous studies have shown that up to 10% of patients use the terms inappropriately to describe situations such as painful sex, structural abnormalities of the penis or even infertility. In addition, the approach to patients describing difficulties in achieving an erection may differ from those men who are not able to maintain tumescence.

General questions

A preliminary enquiry as to why it is a problem and the impact upon the patient's psyche and quality of life can be helpful. It is possible to quantify the severity of ED using subjective validated questionnaires such as the International Index of Erectile Function (IIEF) (see Table 4.1). This is a fairly simple questionnaire to use and offers the opportunity to assess the response to treatment, although it focuses predominantly upon the erectile response rather than quality of life issues. Moreover, an understanding of the partner's attitude to the problem can be enlightening and, wherever possible, the partner should be encouraged to attend the consultation as well. This overview may dictate the subsequent approach by the HCP and in a number of instances it may become clear that no specific treatment is required.

Table 4.1 International Index of Erectile Function (IIEF) domain score

IIEF domain score	Score range
Over the past 4 weeks, how often were you able to get an erection during sexual activity?	0–5
Over the past 4 weeks, when you had erections with sexual stimulation, how often were your erections hard enough for penetration?	0–5
Over the past 4 weeks, when you attempted sexual intercourse, how often were you able to penetrate (enter) your partner?	0–5
Over the past 4 weeks, during sexual intercourse, how difficult was it to maintain your erection after you had penetrated (entered) your partner?	0–5
Over the past 4 weeks, during sexual intercourse, how difficult was it to maintain your erection to completion of intercourse?	0–5
Over the past 4 weeks, how do you rate your confidence that you can keep your erection?	1–5
Total range	1–30*

*A higher score equates with better erectile function.

Speed of onset of ED

Most patients with a predominant psychological aetiology to their ED report a sudden onset to the problem which can often be linked to a stressful life event. It may also be intermittent. Conversely, many patients with organic aetiology present with a slow insidious onset over many months and its development is complete.

The presence of spontaneous erections

Most men experience several spontaneous erections per day, usually at night-time during REM sleep and unrelated to external stimuli. It is assumed (although not proven) that the neural pathway facilitating spontaneous erections is no different from tumescence achieved through sexual arousal. Thus, enquiring about the presence of spontaneous erections may suggest a psychological cause if they are unaffected. The presence of spontaneous erections and rapid speed of onset (and vice versa) are occasionally associated with organic disease and therefore are not always discriminatory symptoms.

Medical history

This should focus upon several key areas reflecting the common causative factors of ED as well as associated pathological conditions.

Vascular

Enquiry about the presence or symptoms of vascular disorders is mandatory. This should include the presence of macrovascular disease (ischaemic heart disease, cerebrovascular disease and peripheral vascular disease), diabetes mellitus and hypertension. In patients with diabetes, the presence of microvascular complications (retinopathy, neuropathy or nephropathy) should be sought. Patients should also be assessed for other risk factors of vascular disease, for instance smoking habits, dyslipidaemia, and a premature family history of vascular disease. The value of this assessment is several-fold:

- There is a strong association between ED and systemic vascular disease and diabetes. ED has also been shown in some research to be an independent risk factor for coronary disease. Thus the presence of ED may herald these hitherto undiscovered conditions.

- Cardiovascular 'fitness' for sex can be determined (see Chapter 5).
- The presence of vascular disease elsewhere may suggest that vascular insufficiency (either atherosclerosis or endothelial dysfunction) is implicated in the development of ED.
- The choice of treatment options may be influenced by the presence of vascular disease, in particular angina.

Neurological

Given the common pathway (S2, S3, S4) of innervation to the bladder and penis, bladder symptoms may indicate a neurological cause of ED. The presence of other motor or sensory symptoms may relate to neurological disease elsewhere, e.g. cerebrovascular disease or demyelination. An autonomic neuropathy affecting the parasympathetic nervous system, particularly in diabetes, is a frequent precipitant of ED and the patient may report other manifestations such as postural hypotension, gustatory sweating or diarrhoea.

Endocrine

Symptoms that suggest hypogonadism (loss of secondary sexual characteristics, reduced libido) should be sought as well as hyperprolactinaemia (usually hypogonadal symptoms associated with gynaecomastia and possibly raised intracranial pressure) and thyroid disorders.

General health

A previous history of prostate disease associated with its treatment (radical or transurethral prostatectomy, or radiotherapy) may be implicated in the development of ED, often through neurovascular damage. Any transient acute illness may be associated with the development of ED. This includes sepsis, acute metabolic disturbances, for example diabetic ketoacidosis, or an acute myocardial infarction. There is often a strong psychological component to its development and in many cases, it spontaneously improves with time.

Drug history

Obtaining an accurate drug history (prescribed and over-the-counter drugs, including alcohol) is required. In the first instance this may identify a drug that has been associated with the development of ED (see Tables 3.3 and 3.4). Next, it is important to determine the temporal relationship between a potential causative drug and the development of ED. In most instances an offending drug has been started within the previous 2 weeks. Stopping listed drugs that the patient has been taking for many years almost never resolves the problem (see Chapter 10).

Psychological effects

It may become evident that a specific life event precipitated the onset of ED or that there is a strong psychological overlay compounding a probable organic aetiology. If time allows, it is helpful to assess several key areas, including misconceptions about normal sexual practice, poor self-esteem and self-image, marital disharmony and anxiety over sexual performance.

Physical examination

Each HCP needs to determine the extent of physical examination they will offer, dependent upon the expertise of the examiner, and whether they plan to offer treatment themselves or refer to a specialist centre. Advances in clinical services have seen, for instance, the development of specialist nurses managing ED, which has been welcomed. Adequate provision for physical assessment needs to be incorporated into the management strategy for patients with ED, which may involve a parallel physical examination by a doctor if this is beyond the remit of the specialist nurse. Evidence of disease elsewhere, for example cardiovascular or neurological disease, may suggest that abnormalities of these systems are linked to the development of ED. The following aspects of examination need to be considered.

Genitalia

Assessment of the penis is mandatory. It should be recognised that in many cases of ED where the primary abnormality is altered smooth muscle relaxation or impaired blood supply within the penis, there may be no visible abnormalities of the penis itself. However, the glans penis may show evidence of balanitis and is associated with a greater incidence of diabetes mellitus. Physical abnormalities may be evident, such as fibrotic plaques within the penile shaft – indicative of Peyronie's disease. Phimosis may be observed. Examination of the testes may reveal reduced testicular volume consistent with hypogonadism. Large epididymal cysts, hydrocoeles or varicocoeles may physically interfere with sexual function or be associated with pain on intercourse or continuous pain. Other signs, less commonly assessed, include palpating each cavernosal artery, thereby indirectly assessing blood flow to the penis, testing sensation over the penis and eliciting the bulbocavernosal reflex which may be impaired in patients with an autonomic neuropathy. The latter test examines S2, S3 and S4 innervation and results in contraction of the anal sphincter as a normal response to pinching the glans penis.

Cardiovascular examination

Assessment should be made for the presence of ischaemic heart disease, cerebrovascular disease (for example carotid bruits) and peripheral vascular disease (skin nutrition, capillary perfusion and the presence of peripheral pulses). Although these findings support the presence of a generalised atherosclerotic process that may be implicated in the development of ED, there are no clinical findings that suggest the presence of endothelial dysfunction, the precursor of atherosclerosis. Blood pressure assessment should be made, including recording of lying and standing measurements. A drop of greater than 20 mmHg systolic and 10 mmHg diastolic is usually considered significant and is consistent with an autonomic neuropathy even in the absence of the patient reporting postural dizziness.

Neurological examination

This may indicate motor or sensory patterns consistent with cerebrovascular disease, demyelination, parkinsonism, peripheral neuropathy or other neurological disorders. Evidence of autonomic neuropathy may be present, which can be assessed by examining the heart rate response to:

- the Valsalva manoeuvre
- standing up
- deep breathing and the blood pressure response to standing up and sustained handgrip.

Endocrine examination

Diabetic microvascular or macrovascular complications may be evident. Pathognomonic small vessel disease may indicate hitherto unsuspected diabetes whilst also supporting a vascular or neurological basis to the patient's ED. Small testes, absence of secondary sexual characteristics, reduced muscle bulk and increased abdominal girth may suggest hypogonadism. Hyperprolactinaemia is associated with gynaecomastia as well as features of hypogonadism. If pituitary pathology is suspected, examination of visual fields may suggest an expansive tumour encroaching upon the optic chiasm (typically a bitemporal hemianopia) and papillodoema may occasionally be present. Altered thyroid metabolism (either thyrotoxicosis or hypothyroidism) may be evident.

Prostate examination

Whilst prostatic disease *per se* is not usually associated with the development of ED, it gives the opportunity to screen for the presence of prostatic cancer, which has a greater prevalence in men over the age of 50 years. Furthermore, its treatment, whether with surgery or radiotherapy, may interrupt normal parasympathetic innervation or blood flow to the penis. Rectal examination also gives an opportunity to assess the bulbocavernosal reflex.

Investigations

The extent of investigation in patients presenting with ED has been extremely variable from practice to practice, ranging from no investigations to very invasive procedures aimed at assessing the competency of blood supply to the penis. In determining which investigations to undertake, it is important to consider two facts:

• Is it necessary to establish the precise diagnosis underlying the patient's ED?
• Does the establishment of a diagnosis offer the prospect of treatment that may hitherto have not been considered?

In many instances the answers to these questions are no, thus negating the need for extensive investigation. Our own practice is to screen for diabetes mellitus in all patients presenting with ED (if not already known), given the observation of a high incidence in this population of patients and the simplicity of screening. Since there is a high false-negative rate associated with urine screening for diabetes, we advocate a fasting plasma

Table 4.2 Further investigations of erectile dysfunction

Penile Doppler studies
Responsiveness to a standard intracavernosal injection
Physiological tests of the autonomic nervous system
Detailed psychosexual assessment
Nocturnal penile rigidity studies
Invasive radiological procedures (penile arteriography or cavernosography)

glucose concentration in the first instance is optimal. Glycated haemoglobin (HbA1c) measurements are a useful long-term indicator of glycaemic control but should not be used to screen for diabetes. We also screen for evidence of hypogonadism, incorporating measurements of total testosterone, luteinising hormone (LH) and follicle-stimulating hormone (FSH) as well as a measure of free testosterone – for example, measuring the sex hormone binding globulin (SHBG) concentration enables the calculation of the free androgen index, an indicator of free ('active') testosterone. We also measure prolactin and thyroid concentrations (free T4, free T3 and TSH concentrations). Some specialists may argue that the detection of these abnormalities are low in the absence of clinical symptoms and signs, and therefore question routine screening.

Other tests that may be employed in investigating ED are summarised in Table 4.2 and are briefly considered below.

Intracavernosal injection testing

Traditionally, intracavernosal injections into the penis (commonly with prostaglandin E1 or papaverine) were used to assess for the presence of significant vascular factors contributing to the patient's ED. Following injection into the penis, tumescence would be expected to occur within 20 minutes if an adequate arterial blood supply and competent venous plexus was present. Lack of erection suggests inadequate blood supply whilst the development of an erection associated with a fairly abrupt detumescence points to leakage within the venous drainage system. We now know the sensitivity and specificity of this test is low in determining the aetiology of ED. However, intracavernosal injections may still be offered in the clinic setting (and often administered by the patient) for assessment of its use as a pharmacological tool to treat ED and whether the patient is capable of self-administration.

Doppler ultrasound of the penis

Traditionally a Doppler ultrasound probe has been used to measure penile systolic blood pressure and compared with systemic systolic blood pressure, usually the brachial artery. A ratio below 0.6 was thought to indicate a vascular aetiology, although the reliability of this test is now disputed. In particular, whilst low ratios may support a vascular cause (high sensitivity), the finding of a near normal ratio does not (low specificity).

Measurement of penile nocturnal rigidity

The presence of nocturnal rigidity can be measured using simple devices such as a snap gauge (Figure 4.1a) or more sophisticated equipment using a penile strain gauge connected to an external recorder (Figure 4.1b). This can be coupled with an oculogram which measures REM sleep. The basis of this test is that most men usually experience nocturnal (physiological) erections during REM sleep. Previous studies have suggested that patients with organic disease have abnormal or no nocturnal erections whilst they are preserved in patients with a psychological basis to their ED. Again, the value of this test is disputed and discrimination between an organic and psychological cause can usually be made by other means. It should also be noted that coexistence of organic and psychological contributory factors is quite common.

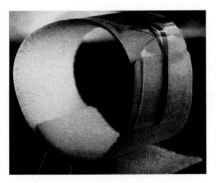

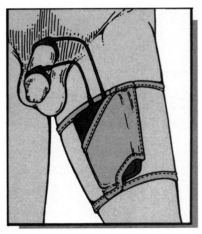

Figure 4.1 (a) Snap gauge. (b) Nocturnal penile tumescence monitoring (plethysmography).

Detailed autonomic nerve testing

Techniques for more detailed analysis of autonomic nerve testing are in abundance. Most examine cardiovascular reflexes employing computer technology to calculate whether responses lie outside the normal reference range. Other tests assess sweat production (the sweat spot test) or papillary dilation. Experimentally, many cases of ED have been linked to abnormal parasympathetic responses but the value of investigating for its presence in clinical practice is limited.

Invasive radiological testing

Penile arteriography is usually only undertaken in specialist centres where patients may be considered for reconstructive arterial surgery. Following the introduction of an intracavernosal smooth muscle relaxant such as prostaglandin E1, the arterial circulation is assessed after catheterisation of the femoral artery, which enables the penile vasculature to be examined in detail.

Cavernosography may be considered by specialists centres if venous leakage is suspected that may be amenable to venous ligation. This technique involves the simultaneous infusion of fluid (usually saline) into the penile body whilst introducing contrast media into the penile vasculature which may demonstrate significant venous return during tumescence.

Key points

- A careful history and examination may indicate a likely organic or psychological cause of ED, or both.
- Assessment for the presence or risk of cardiovascular disease and diabetes mellitus is important since they commonly coexist.
- Extensive investigation is rarely required since the outcome of these tests does not usually influence subsequent treatment choice.
- Further investigations are generally best determined on an individual basis related to clinical suspicion and if their presence would alter the clinical management of ED.

Further reading

Alexander WD, Cummings MH. (1996) Erectile dysfunction and its treatment. In: Shaw KM (ed.), *Diabetic Complications*. Chichester: John Wiley and Sons.

Buvat J, Lemaire A. (1997) Endocrine screening in 1033 men with erectile dysfunction: clinical significance and cost-effective strategy. *Journal of Urology* **158**, 1764–7.

Ewing DJ, Martyn CN, Young RJ, Clarke BF. (1985) The value of cardiovascular autonomic function tests. *Diabetes Care* **8**, 491–8.

Queral LA, Whitehouse WM, Flinn WR, Zains CK, Bergan JJ, Yao JST. (1979) Pelvic haemodynamics after aortoiliac reconstruction. *Surgery* **86**, 799–803.

Rosen RC, Riley A, Wagner G, Osterloh H, Kirkpatrick J, Mishra A. (1997) The International Index of of Erectile Function (IIEF): a multidimensional scale for assessment of erectile dysfunction. *Urology* **49**, 822–30.

5 WHAT PRACTICAL ISSUES SHOULD I CONSIDER BEFORE OFFERING TREATMENT?

Cardiovascular 'fitness'

There are often misconceptions about the level of exertion associated with sexual activity. This has been evaluated in research studies and found to be no more strenuous than lifting and carrying objects weighing between 9 and 20 kg or playing golf. These studies employ the units known as the metabolic equivalent of the task (MET) which enables the consumption of oxygen per task according to body weight to be assigned and compared across a range of physical activities.

It has been demonstrated that sexual intercourse with a longstanding partner is equivalent to between 2–3 METs with an upper range of 4–5 METs during more vigorous activity. This compares with METs for other activities shown in Table 5.1. Thus, for patients with established angina, it is possible to ascertain whether sexual activity is likely to be safe or precipitate undesired chest pain by comparison with other non-sexual activities. This explanation can also be helpful in reducing performance anxiety in some patients who may have concerns about resuming sexual activity after myocardial infarction (MI). It has been estimated that sexual activity may trigger an MI approximately 30 chances per million per hour in the 2-hour period following sexual activity and is associated with the development of an MI in less than 1% of cases. Thus, for the majority of cardiac patients, it is possible to reassure them (and the HCP) that sexual activity is unlikely to precipitate a major cardiac event.

Previous consensus guidelines by Jackson et al. (1999) have been helpful in developing a framework for stratifying patients at cardiovascular risk following a significant absence from sexual activity. Patients are classified into three risk groups (low, intermediate and high risk), which enables the HCP to determine whether it is reasonable to proceed to management of ED without delay or whether further cardiovascular evaluation is required (see Table 5.2).

Table 5.1 MET equivalents*

Daily activity	MET score
Sexual intercourse with longstanding partner:	
Lower range ('normal')	2–3
Upper range ('vigorous activity')	5–6
Lifting and carrying objects (9–20 kg)	4–5
Light housework (e.g. ironing or polishing)	2–4
Heavy housework (e.g. making beds, scrubbing floors)	3–6
DIY work	4–5
Walking 1 mile on the flat within 20 minutes	3–4
Golf	4–5

*From Wilson PK, Farday PS, Froelicher V (eds) (1981) *Cardiac Rehabilitation: Adult Fitness and Exercise Testing*, pp. 333–53. Philadelphia: Lea and Fabiger.

Underlying disorders requiring specific treatment or affecting treatment choice

There are a number of conditions or their treatment that may affect management strategies. A few important examples are briefly illustrated below.

Cardiovascular disease

Cardiovascular disease needs to be assessed and managed appropriately before embarking upon treatment for ED (see above). Patients on nitrate therapy or nicorandil should not use phosphodiesterase type 5 (PDE5) inhibitors (see Chapter 7) whilst patients on warfarin should avoid intraurethral pellets or intracavernosal injections (see Chapter 8) and vacuum devices (see Chapter 9) because of the increased risk of penile bleeding and haematoma.

Diabetes mellitus

Diabetes mellitus needs to be assessed for and if present, a search made for the presence of other concomitant microvascular or macrovascular complications that may need treatment. Whilst the treatment options may be similar to the non-diabetic population, the effectiveness of the therapeutic intervention may be reduced (see Chapter 10).

Table 5.2 Approach to the management of ED according to cardiovascular risk

Grading of risk	CV status at presentation	Recommendation for the management of ED
Low risk	Controlled hypertension	Manage ED within primary care setting
	Asymptomatic ≤3 risk factors for CAD	Review treatment options with patient and partner (where possible)
	Mild valvular disease Mild stable angina Post successful revascularisation	
Intermediate risk	Recent MI or CVA (within 6 weeks)	Specialised evaluation recommended (for example exercise testing or echocardiography)
	≥3 risk factors for CAD	Place patient in high or low group upon outcome of testing
	LVD, CHF (New York Heart Association class I, II) Murmur of unknown cause Moderate stable angina	
High risk	Unstable or refractory angina	Refer for specialised cardiac evaluation and management
	Uncontrolled hypertension (systolic BP >180 mmHg)	Treatment for ED to be deferred until cardiac condition stabilised and/or specialist evaluation completed
	CHF (New York Heart Association class III, IV) Recent MI or CVA (within last 14 days) High risk arrhythmias Hypertrophic cardiomyopathy Moderate/severe valvular disease	

CAD, coronary artery disease; CHF, chronic heart failure; CV, cardiovascular; CVA, cardiovascular accident; LVD, left ventricular dysfunction.

Hypogonadism, hyperprolactinaemia and thyroid disease

Resolution of the metabolic abnormalities hypogonadism, hyperprolactinaemia and thyroid disease (see Chapter 10), unlike treating diabetes, are usually associated with improvement in ED. However, for some patients regaining tumescence can be delayed, most commonly related to residual performance anxiety. In these patients psychosexual support or temporary drug intervention can help restore potency.

Primary penile abnormalities

ED may resolve with correction of primary penile abnormalities *per se* without the need for further specific intervention (see Chapter 9).

Psychological or psychiatric disorders associated with ED

Psychological or psychiatric disorders associated with ED are best dealt with by psychosexual counsellors or psychiatrists. Some patients may refuse these services because of the stigma associated with this course of action. Careful assessment may identify patients who may benefit from physical treatments for ED (for example, where it is clear that ED is a major contributor to the patient's depression).

Impact upon relationships

Whilst in most relationships the return of potency is greeted with happiness, this is not always the case. It cannot be stressed enough the importance of assessing the partner's view of the problem, ideally directly at the consultation if they attend. Resuming sexual relationships can be an undesired event for some females and may reflect underlying anxiety or physical problems such as vaginismus or predisposition to cystitis.

Department of Health guidance on the treatment of ED

Treatment of ED continues to be supported by the Department of Health (DoH) in the UK following guidance in 1999 (see Table 5.3). Prior to this document, there had been little national guidance on the treatment of ED and this may have reflected little need, given the sparseness of ad hoc ED

Table 5.3 Summary of Department of Health Guidelines (1999) for prescribing in ED

All drugs used for the treatment of ED classified under Schedule 2, previously Schedule 11 (restricted availability)
Eligible groups of medical conditions for treatment of ED: diabetes mellitus, all patients with prostate cancer, spinal cord injury, demyelination, renal failure, severe pelvic injury, spina bifida, polio, Parkinson's disease, single gene neurological disease
ED causing 'severe distress' (confirmed by a hospital consultant)
Patients already receiving treatment for ED before 14/9/98 (irrespective of the aetiology)

services, often using unlicensed preparations in the treatment of ED. With the licensing and potential demand for PDE5 inhibitors, it was recognised that guidance for HCPs was required, which identified groups of patients that were eligible for treatment under the state health system (NHS), listed in Table 5.3. It was recommended that NHS scripts should be limited to no more than one treatment per week for ED and further demand would require patients to finance private prescriptions. Subsequently, it has been shown that the treatment of ED is affordable (see Chapter 1) and it is hoped the DoH will remove the capping of prescriptions and patient groups under the state health system. It would make sense to determine treatment based upon the severity of ED and its impact upon the patient's quality of life rather than the nature of the underlying condition.

Primary care – specialist care interface

The introduction of PDE5 inhibitors has led to a shift of management towards primary care with specialist care often reserved for patients in whom oral therapy is contraindicated or in non-responders. In many instances this has required an uplift in skills within primary care to ensure patients are properly assessed and counselled about their treatment. It has been observed that failure of oral therapy, for instance, may be associated with inappropriate or ignored advice in up to one-third of non-responders. Fortunately, there is only a relative minority of patients who do not respond to oral treatment and it is essential that there is an opportunity for patients to be offered second-line treatment options. These treatments are often invasive or are time consuming to explain and discuss with the patients. Few primary care centres are able to offer these services, requiring specialist referral, usually to departments of urology, diabetes or sexual medicine, or to psychosexual counsellors.

Key points

- Practical advice can determine the safeness of sexual activity by comparing its energy expenditure (using METs) with other physical activities.
- Practical guidelines also exist to enable the HCP to determine the level of cardiac risk for resuming sexual activity in the individual with ED and whether further cardiac evaluation and treatment may be required first.
- Consideration to medical conditions (such as cardiac disease, diabetes mellitus, endocrine abnormalities, penile abnormalities, concomitant drug therapy) or psychological disorders, as well as the views of the partner, need to be considered prior to treatment of ED to ensure the most effective and safest mode of treatment is offered.
- Treatment of ED is affordable and warranted under the NHS.
- HCPs need to be aware of treatment options and referral routes for all treatment modalities that may be offered to the patient.

References and further reading

Central Office of Information Health (1999) *Impotence Consultation Document.* Number 0274.

De Busk R, Drory Y, Goldstein I, Jackson G. (2000) Management of sexual dysfunction in patients with cardiovascular disease: recommendations of the Princeton Consensus Panel. *American Journal of Cardiology* **86**, 175–81.

Jackson G, Betteridge J, Dean J, Hall R, Holdright D, Holmes S, Kirby M, Riley A, Sever P. (1999) A systematic approach to erectile dysfunction in the cardiovascular patient: a consensus statement. *International Journal of Clinical Practice* **53**, 445–51.

Moller J, Ahlbom A, Hulting J. (2001) Sexual activity as a trigger of myocardial infarction. The case cross-over analysis in the Stockholm Heart Epidemiology Programme (SHEP). *Heart* **86**, 376–90.

Muller JE, Mittleman MA, Maclure M. (1996) Triggering myocardial infarction by sexual activity. *Journal of the American Medical Association* **276**, 1405–9.

6 MANAGEMENT ALGORITHM

In the management of ED, as with other conditions, it is always helpful to have a management strategy in place. A suggested algorithm for the treatment of ED is shown in Figure 6.1, although this may be adapted according to local provision and guidelines. At each stage it is important to ascertain the HCP responsible for a given step in the algorithm. Local knowledge of the provision of specialist ED care facilitates the most appropriate referral route if required. Each of the treatment options are covered in more detail in the following chapters.

Figure 6.1 (overleaf) indicates that there are few options that will result in spontaneous resolution of the patient's ED. However, recent evidence has demonstrated that weight loss (in this study, a mean loss of 15 kg equivalent to 14.5% of original body weight) was associated with improved erections and a concomitant improvement in endothelial dysfunction (a known cause of ED) and vascular inflammation.

Further reading

Esposito K, Giugliano F, Di Palo C, Giugliano G, Marfella R, D'Andrea F, D'Armiento M, Giugliano D. (2004) Effect of lifestyle changes on erectile dysfunction in obese men. *Journal of the American Medical Association* **291**(24), 2978–84.

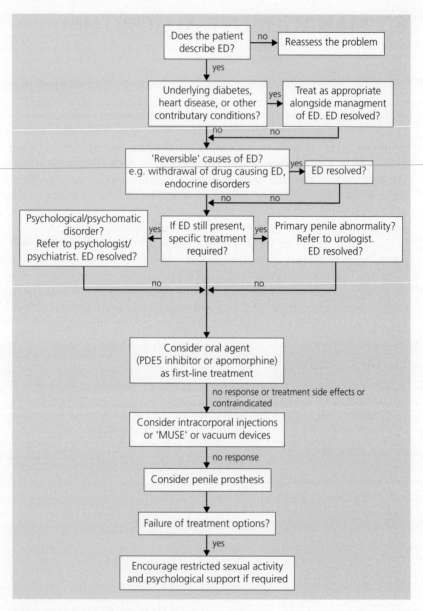

Figure 6.1 Algorithm for the treatment of ED.

7 ORAL THERAPY: WHEN AND HOW?

Until 1998 there was little that could be offered as effective oral therapy for ED. At that time, the most commonly used agent was yohimbine. This drug was thought to mediate its effect through its competitive antagonist action on alpha-adrenoreceptors within the brain, suggesting that it enhanced libido. Clinical trials as well as patient experience have indicated that yohimbine has not been an effective agent for treating ED and yohimbine was never licensed for use within the UK.

In 1998, the introduction of phosphodiesterase type 5 (PDE5) inhibitors revolutionised almost overnight the management of ED in several ways. First, the media attention associated with its release meant that the public and HCPs became more accustomed to talking about the subject whereas previously it was considered by many to be a taboo subject. Patients became much more knowledgeable about ED, and national advice centres became available as it widely became known that effective non-invasive treatment was available for the treatment of ED. Moreover, there was a shift towards more treatment being offered for ED in the primary care setting without time delays seeking specialist care evaluation. This has resulted in many more patients seeking advice for the treatment of ED, and Department of Health guidelines supporting the use of PDE5 inhibitors.

PDE5 inhibitors

Initially evaluated for the treatment of angina, this class of drugs was found to be very effective in restoring potency in men with ED. Currently three oral agents are available within the UK. They are sildenafil (Viagra, 25–100 mg) marketed by Pfizer Pharmaceuticals, tadalafil (Cialis, 10–20 mg) marketed by Eli Lilly Pharmaceuticals, and vardenafil (Levitra, 5–20 mg) marketed by Bayer Pharmaceuticals. The mechanism of action of these drugs is to facilitate smooth muscle relaxation within the penis through enhancing the availability of cyclic GMP by reducing its rate of breakdown (see Figures 2.1 and 7.1).

43

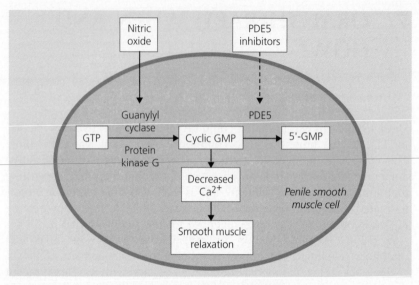

Figure 7.1 Mechanism of action of PDE5 inhibitors.

Pharmacokinetic properties

The pharmacokinetic properties of sildenafil and vardenafil are similar, reflecting little difference in their chemical structure. Conversely, the significant difference in chemical structure of tadalafil confers contrasting pharmacokinetic properties (see Table 7.1). The rapid absorption across the digestive tract of all three agents mean that they are effective usually within 30 minutes. However, absorption of tadalafil appears to be unaffected by food (especially fatty food) in contrast to sildenafil and vardenafil (see Table 7.1). In addition, the half life of tadalafil (17.5 hours) is much greater than for sildenafil or vardenafil (approximately 4 hours for both). This extended period of therapeutic responsiveness can allow men to choose when to attempt intercourse for up to 36 hours after taking tadalafil compared with about 4 hours for sildenafil or vardenafil.

Table 7.1 The pharmacokinetic properties of the three oral PDE5 inhibitors after a single dose

Parameter	Sildenafil	Tadalafil	Vardenafil
Dose (mg)	100	20	20
Bioavailability (%)	41	NK	15
Change in C_{max} after fatty food (%)*	↓ 29%	↔	↓ 20%
T_{max} (h)	0.8	2.0	0.66
Half-life (h)	3.7	17.5	4.4

*After a standardised fatty meal. C_{max}, maximal plasma concentration; T_{max}, time to maximum concentration; NK, not known.

Efficacy

There is now a large body of evidence to support the effectiveness of all three PDE5 inhibitors in the treatment of ED. Attempts have been made to compare the effectiveness of these drugs in the absence of head-to-head trials. Such comparisons are fraught with difficulties for many reasons. First, the subjective scales used to assess the response to ED may differ. Second, the characteristics of the patients being evaluated may be very different and be affected by the severity of ED and the underlying cause. It is recognised also that patients who are treatment naïve may well respond better initially than those patients who have been previously treated for ED. Finally, the doses of PDE5 inhibitors used in clinical trials may not allow fair comparisons. Broadly speaking, however, their efficacy appears to be similar, with perhaps four out of five patients responding to treatment in the general population. This figure is consistently reduced (approximately three out of five patients) in patients with underlying diabetes mellitus. The efficacy and tolerability of this class of drugs have led to their use as first-line agents in patients requiring treatment for ED.

Tolerability

This class of drugs is generally very well tolerated and very few patients experience side-effects which necessitate withdrawing the drug. Side-effects can be divided into those that are class specific and those unique to the individual drug. The class-specific side-effects are listed in Table 7.2 and often are mild and transient. It is thought they arise through

45

Table 7.2 Class side-effects of PDE5 inhibitors

Headaches
Dyspepsia
Flushing
Dizziness
Nasal congestion

inhibition of PDE5 in other smooth muscle beds, leading to vasodilation in tissues such as the nasal cavities and brain. This systemic vasodilatory response through inhibition of PDE5 is thought to explain any associated hypotension and has led to the concomitant use of nitrate therapy (including sublingual nitrates) and nicorandil being contraindicated.

Unique side-effects relate to the individual drug's ability to affect other phosphodiesterase enzymes. For instance, the inhibition of PDE6 isoenzyme (found in the rod and cone cells of the retina) by sildenafil and vardenafil may lead to minor visual disturbances, often reported as a transient blue-green haze in the periphery of vision. Conversely, tadalafil has been shown to inhibit PDE11 isoenzyme found in skeletal muscle and testes. This may explain the slightly greater incidence of mild back pain associated with tadalafil use, although this is speculative in the absence of supportive clinical data. Given the finding of PDE11 in the testes, subsequent studies have confirmed no relevant affects of tadalafil on spermatogenesis in humans nor effects on reproductive hormone metabolism.

A large body of evidence now exists to show that use of the oral PDE5 inhibitors is not associated with a greater risk of cardiovascular disease.

Practical tips on the use of PDE5 inhibitors

It is important that patients understand how this class of drugs promotes an erection. Many patients report that the use of these drugs did not result in erection and were unaware that they prime the penis (a 'peripheral conditioner') to be more receptive to sexual arousal. Patients also need to be aware of the 'window of opportunity' following ingestion to maximise the drug's potential. Moreover, research has shown that the response rate is lower following the first use of a PDE5 inhibitor

Table 7.3 *Side-effects of sublingual apomorphine*

Nausea
Headaches
Dyspepsia
Dizziness
Yawning
Drowsiness
Rhinitis and pharyngitis
Rarely, syncope

compared with subsequent dosing. It is our own practice to advise patients to try a specific dose on at least six occasions to gauge its effectiveness. The effectiveness of these drugs is greatest at the higher range, so simply titrating doses may result in a positive outcome compared with lower doses. Food intake prior to PDE5 inhibitor ingestion may also reduce the effectiveness of sildenafil and vardenafil (see above). Finally, PDE5 inhibitors have no known beneficial effects in patients with normal erectile function.

Apomorphine

Traditionally, apomorphine has been used to treat parkinsonism but the discovery that it promoted erections led to studies evaluating its treatment for ED in man. The effects of this drug are thought to be through its ability to stimulate dopamine (D2) receptors within the hypothalamic and limbic neural pathways, thereby enhancing arousal. Apomorphine hydrochloride (Uprima, 2–3 mg) is licensed within the UK for the treatment of ED and is marketed by Abbott Laboratories as a sublingual preparation.

The study evidence compared with the PDE5 inhibitors is limited but, overall, it would appear that approximately up to 45% of patients may respond in the general population and again the effectiveness is reduced in patients with diabetes mellitus. This success rate is less than seen with PDE5 inhibitors and its use in clinical practice has often been for patients who have not responded or have had side-effects with the latter class of drugs. In particular, one potential use of apomorphine may be in patients with stable heart disease who require the use of nitrates or nicorandil, in whom PDE5 inhibitors are contraindicated.

The side-effects of apomorphine are shown in Table 7.3. Higher doses of apomorphine cause a paradoxical decrease in efficacy and are associated with a much higher incidence of side-effects, particularly nausea. Although the combination of PDE5 inhibitors and apomorphine may be attractive given their synergistic modes of action, there are no published studies to date that have evaluated this dual approach.

Key points

- Oral PDE5 inhibitors have revolutionised the approach to management of ED and, in most cases requiring treatment, represent the first-line approach.
- Three commercially available agents are available (sildenafil, tadalafil and vardenafil).
- The efficacy of these three drugs is similar although the pharmacokinetic profiles differ, resulting in differing durations of action and interaction with food.
- Side-effects are infrequent, mild and often transient, related to the inhibition of PDE5 in other smooth muscle beds or other PDE isoenzymes.
- An alternative to PDE5 inhibitors is sublingual apomorphine, although its effectiveness, by comparison, is reduced.

Further reading

Eardley I, Cartledge J. (2002) Tadalafil (Cialis) for men with erectile dysfunction. *International Journal of Clinical Practice* **56**, 300–4.
Goldstein I, Lue TF, Padma-Nathan H, Rosen RC, Steers WD, Wicker PA. (1988) Oral sildenafil in the treatment of erectile dysfunction. Sildenafil Study Group. *New England Journal of Medicine* **338**, 1397–404.
Hellstrom WJG, Overstreet JW, Yu A, Saikali K, Shen W, Beasley Jr CM, Watkins VS. (2003) Tadalafil has no detrimental effect on human spermatogenesis or reproductive hormones. *Journal of Urology* **170**, 887–91.
Morales A, Gingell C, Collins M. (1998) Clinical safety of oral sildenafil citrate (Viagra) in the treatment of erectile dysfunction. *International Journal of Impotence Research* **10**, 69–74.

Porst H, Rosen R, Padma-Nathan H. (2001) The efficacy and tolerability of vardenafil, a new, oral, selective phosphodiesterase type 5 inhibitor, in patients with erectile dysfunction: the first at-home clinical trial. *International Journal of Impotence Research* **13**, 192–9.

Stief C, Padley RJ, Perdok RJ, Sleep DJ. (2002) Cross-study review of the clinical efficacy of apomorphine SL 2 and 3 mg: pooled data from three placebo-controlled, fixed-dose crossover studies. *European Journal of Urology* **1**, 12–20.

50

8 INVASIVE PHARMACOLOGICAL THERAPY: WHEN AND HOW?

Intracorporal self-injection therapy

Until the introduction of oral PDE5 inhibitors, penile injections (intra-corporal self-injection therapy, ICSIT) remained the mainstay of treatment for most patients with ED. The range of injectable agents used is shown in Table 8.1 and all promote smooth muscle relaxation within the corpus cavernosum. For many years within the UK papaverine was used as an unlicensed preparation. The introduction of a licensed injectable drug, prostaglandin E1 (PGE1) has largely replaced this practice and has been found to be more effective than papaverine and less commonly associated with the development of priapism. Whilst oral PDE5 inhibitors are the first line of treatment, ICSIT is perhaps the most common alternative successful treatment strategy employed.

Table 8.1 Drugs used for intracorporal injections in the treatment of ED

Drug	Comment
Prostaglandin E1 (PGE1)*	Stimulates cyclic AMP Licensed for use within the UK
Papaverine*	Non-specific phosphodiesterase inhibitor Not licensed for use within the UK
Phentolamine*	Non-specific alpha-adrenergic receptor blocker Ineffective as single agent Not licensed for use within the UK
Moxisylyte	Specific alpha-1-adrenergic receptor blocker Withdrawn from the UK market but available elsewhere in Europe
Vasoactive intestinal polypeptide (VIP)	Stimulates cyclic AMP Not currently licensed for use within the UK but available elsewhere in Europe

*Used by some specialist centres as a triple mixture for intracorporal injection.

51

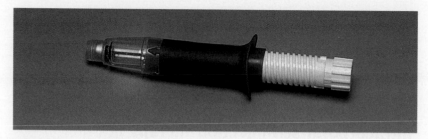

Figure 8.1 Intracorporal delivery of PGE1 using a single use Caverject device.

Mechanism of action

Chapter 2 has discussed the mechanisms by which the important process of smooth muscle relaxation is achieved within the penis, allowing pooling of blood within the sinusoid lakes of the penile tissue facilitating tumescence. It is perhaps not surprising, therefore, that each of the drugs used as ICSIT ultimately leads to a drop in intracellular calcium by enhancing the availability of cyclic AMP or cyclic GMP (see Figure 2.4). An important difference compared with oral PDE5 inhibitors is they can promote smooth muscle relaxation in the absence of enhanced libido.

The technique of ICSIT

Teaching patients to use ICSIT is time consuming. Few primary care HCPs offer this treatment, but it is important to be aware of this treatment modality and a source of referral to specialist centres. In doing so, it is possible to offer an optimistic approach to patients who have not responded to oral therapy. Specialist centres may include urology departments, diabetes centres, departments of sexual medicine, psychosexual counsellors and some specialist centres within primary care run usually by GPs with an interest in ED.

The approach to teaching ICSIT may vary between specialist centres and from patient to patient. This may range from observing patients self-injecting a test dose at their first visit (thereby assessing their technique rather than response) to the HCP administering the injection at a dose designed to induce an erection. Both approaches have their merits. The former option gives the patient confidence that they can self-inject whilst the latter approach in most incidences provides confidence that the treatment can facilitate tumescence. Whichever technique is employed, the reassuring finding is that most patients find ICSIT less uncomfortable to administer than they may have previously perceived. It should be noted that initial lack of response to a 'high' test dose of ICSIT does not necessarily imply failure since patients may often respond to subsequent dosing, particularly in more relaxed environ-ments than a hospital bed or out-patient setting.

PGE1 is available in two forms within the UK, Caverject (Pharmacia, 2.5–60 mcg) and Viridal Duo (Schwarz, 2.5–40 mcg). In view of the instability in solution, PGE1 is provided in powder form within a dual chamber cartridge that is mixed with the diluent using a single appli-cator device immediately before injection (see Figure 8.1). The other preparations used (for example, papaverine or the triple mix of PGE1, papaverine and phentolamine) require the use of a standard needle and syringe technique and are less convenient. It is important that the

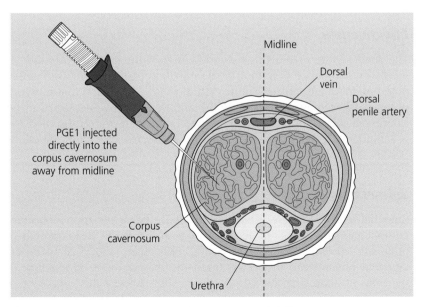

Figure 8.2   Correct injection site for intracorporal delivery.

53

technique is adequately explained to the patient, usually both verbally and through written instructions. This may utilise the literature and diagrams provided by the manufacturers, although in many specialist centres adapted information leaflets are also provided. Whilst consent forms are not strictly necessary with PGE1, some centres still use them, given the invasive nature of the technique, to ensure the patient feels fully conversant with the technique. Consent forms should be mandatory for patients using a non-licensed preparation. The usual technique employs patients using a titration technique, usually starting with 2.5–5 mcg of PGE1, increasing in increments of 5–10 mcg until a desired response is achieved. This is usually defined as an erection suitable for sexual intercourse that lasts no longer than 1 hour. The most appropriate site of injection is within the side of the shaft of the penis (see Figure 8.2), following which the patient should briefly gently massage the penis and walk around the room to facilitate an effective response. In most cases, an erection will develop within 10–15 minutes. Injections should not be repeated within 24 hours or excessive incremental increases be employed, since this exponentially increases the risk of priapism.

Effectiveness

The success rate of ICSIT is extremely high if the correct technique is used with avoidance of inappropriate injection sites and excessive doses that may induce priapism. Clinical studies have suggested that nine out of ten patients may respond to PGE1 and this success rate seems to be similar in diabetic patients. The rate-limiting factor is usually the psychological barrier associated with the process of penile injections *per se* or unacceptable side-effects.

Side-effects

Potential side-effects are listed in Table 8.2. By far the most important complication that patients need to be aware of is the development of priapism – prolonged erections lasting more than 4 hours. It is important that patients are instructed upon the management of priapism at the time of educating them in the use of ICSIT since this represents a medical emergency. Priapism has been associated with permanent hypoxic damage to the corpus cavernosum.

54

Table 8.2 Side-effects of intracorporal injections

Penile bruising (in up to 25% of cases)
Penile pain (in up to 30% of cases)
Priapism
Dizziness, hypotension and syncope
Fibrosis and scarring at the injection site
Local damage (urethra or dorsal vein) with inappropriate injection site
Infection

Priapism

Fortunately, the incidence of priapism is extremely low with PDE1 when used appropriately (<0.1% of all injections). Should it develop, there are a few simple measures that patients can take to see if they can induce detumescence. They can:

- attempt to reduce penile blood flow by the application of ice packs (or similar frozen objects) around the penis
- exercise to promote enhanced blood flow in the lower limbs
- make further attempts at sexual intercourse.

Where these options fail, it is important the patient attends an emergency centre for specialist help. In the first instance, repeated aspiration of 50 ml aliquots of blood directly from the corpus cavernosum following the introduction of a butterfly needle may help. If there is no response, a selective alpha-1-adrenergic agent (usually phenylephrine, starting dose 200 mcg) may be used and repeated if necessary. These steps are largely successful in reversing priapism and it is very rare to necessitate progressing to surgical intervention using a shunt procedure.

Transurethral therapy

It is recognised that the urethral lining facilitates access of substances, introduced into the urethra, to the corpus cavernosum through the local penile circulation. This observation has led to the development of intraurethral pellets of PGE1 which are used to treat ED. The only licensed preparation available within the UK is MUSE (Medicated Urethral System for Erection) manufactured by Meda (dose range 125–1000 mcg). The larger dose range of PGE1 compared with ICSIT reflects the need to ensure adequate drug availability is achieved within the penile smooth muscle via this indirect route of administration.

Application of MUSE

As with ICSIT, it is imperative that patients are fully instructed about the use of MUSE by the HCP. Many specialists will observe the patient introducing an intraurethral pellet as a test dose in the first instance to ensure the technique is correct. The manufacturer's instructions are helpful and may be supplemented by local guidelines. It is advantageous if patients micturate before pellet insertion since it is thought that residual urine drops may more rapidly dissolve the pellet. The stem of the MUSE device is then placed into the urethra and depression of the applicator button ejects the pellet into the urethra (see Figure 8.3). Massaging the penis helps to disperse the PGE1 and successful erections can be observed within 10–15 minutes. Dose titration is usually required as for ICSIT and no more than one application should be applied per 24-hour period even in the event of initial lack of response. In some patients, a partial response may be improved by the simultaneous use of a constriction ring placed around the base of the penis.

Effectiveness

The effectiveness in clinical trials has indicated that two out of three patients may respond in the general population regardless of aetiology.

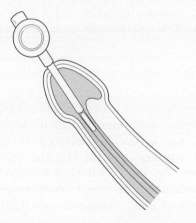

Figure 8.3   Application of 'MUSE'.

56

Table 8.3 Side-effects of transurethral alprostadil ('MUSE')

Penile pain (in up to 30% of cases or more)
Dizziness, hypotension and syncope
Urethral trauma and occasional bleeding

Subsequent clinical experience in our centre and elsewhere suggests that even after optimum dose titration, this figure is lower, which suggests in part that an inadequate dose of PGE1 is reaching the corpus cavernosum. A successful response is also hindered by a high frequency of side-effects in patients using MUSE. However, for a number of men with ED, MUSE represents a more acceptable approach to ICSIT and may often be tried first.

Side-effects

Reported side-effects are shown in Table 8.3. The most troublesome complication is heterogeneous pain (in up to one-third of patients), either in the penis itself or the upper thighs. Whilst mild in may cases, it may negate a satisfactory response to MUSE. Unlike ICSIT, priapism is virtually non-existent.

Key points

- In patients who fail to respond to first-line treatment with oral PDE5 inhibitors or apomorphine, intracorporal injections or intraurethral pellets of prostaglandin E1 offer an acceptable effective alternative.
- Although primary care HCPs may not be proficient in teaching patients the use of these agents, they should be aware of the principles and local referral routes to specialist centres that offer this service.
- All patients need to be adequately taught by HCPs on the technique of administration, dose titration and potential side-effects. In particular, patients need to know how to manage priapism, an uncommon complication of self-injection therapy.

Further reading

Alexander WD, Cummings MH. (1996) Erectile dysfunction and its treatment. In: Shaw KM (ed.), *Diabetic Complications*. Chichester: John Wiley & Sons.

Linet OI, Ogrinc FG. (1996) Efficacy and safety of intracavernosal alprostadil in men with erectile dysfunction. *New England Journal of Medicine* **334**, 873–7.

Padma-Nathan H, Hellstrom W, Kaiser FE. (1997) Treatment of men with erectile dysfunction with transurethral alprostadil. *New England Journal of Medicine* **36**, 1–7.

Virag R. (1982) Intracavernous injection of papaverine for erectile failure. *Lancet* **2**, 938.

9 ARE THERE ANY ALTERNATIVE APPROACHES TO DRUG THERAPY?

Psychosexual counselling

Psychosexual counselling may be useful in two situations:

- in those patients with ED who have been identified with a clear psychological or psychiatric disorder that has contributed to its development
- in those patients with ED who have an underlying organic cause which is worsened by a secondary psychological component. This combined approach is intuitively believed to be more effective than just employing a pharmacological agent, although it remains unproven in clinical studies.

The extent and type of counselling will depend on the underlying cause and may require psychiatric input to address a more generalised order, or specific psychosexual counselling focusing upon a particular area identified within the sexual history. The history may identify predisposing factors (for example issues within the patient's family environment and upbringing), precipitating factors (for example life events, both physical and psychological) and factors maintaining the impotent state (for example performance anxiety or partner communication issues). This may identify a specific issue that needs to be addressed with the patient or the relationship and/or lead to a more generalised approach such as behavioural therapy. Whilst it may be identified that psychological issues appear to be the predominant problem contributing to the patient's ED, some males resist the offer of psychosexual therapy because of the stigma associated with consulting a counsellor or the partner may be unwilling to attend. In these circumstances it may be appropriate to introduce alternative treatment such as oral PDE5 inhibitors. Improvement in erectile function may overcome some of these psychological issues such as performance anxiety, which allows subsequent withdrawal of drug therapy.

Behavioural therapies

There are numerous techniques employed to restore sexual function, but one of those most commonly used and shown to be successful in clinical studies is the approach of Masters and Johnson (1970). This employs a progressive programme designed to enhance communication in the relationship as well as recognising the desires and concerns of each partner. This form of so-called sensate focusing involves three main stages – non-genital, genital and vaginal containment, with a ban on sexual intercourse until all stages are complete.

- The *non-genital stage* allows caressing and stroking each other's naked body other than the genital areas. It is designed to reintroduce intimacy and closeness yet avoid possible threatening situations that may be posed by genital contact.
- The *genital phase* allows the above process to continue, incorporating genital stimulation through caressing and touching. In many instances tumescence may occur but sexual intercourse should remain prohibited.
- *Vaginal containment* allows vaginal penetration initially without movement, subsequently progressing to full sexual activity leading to ejaculation and climax.

Alternative approaches to behavioural therapy include cognitive therapy (using rational argument to challenge deviant thought processes) or occasionally psychoanalytical therapy (to address previous earlier experiences affecting sexual function).

Vacuum devices

Some males with ED prefer to adopt a non-pharmacological approach and the use of a vacuum device may be appropriate. These devices can now be prescribed under the NHS and offer a cost-effective approach (price range usually approximately £80–300) if deemed acceptable. They are generally unsuitable for patients who do not have a stable relationship and given the rather cumbersome nature of the device, can be off-putting for some men. Many retail sex shops sell cheap versions of vacuum devices (less than £50) but they are generally not robust and suffer from the lack of training in their use, which is essential. Thus the success rate with over-the-counter devices is low.

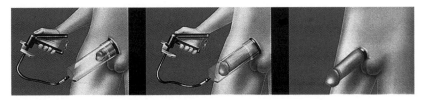

Figure 9.1 Application of a vacuum device.

The use of vacuum devices

Various vacuum devices are available, either manual or battery operated, which employ the same principles. The vacuum cylinder is placed over the penis after a rubber constrictor ring is placed around the proximal end of the cylinder (see Figure 9.1). At the distal end, the cylinder is connected to a pump that, upon activation, induces a vacuum within the cylinder. In consequence, an erection is achieved which is maintained upon removal of the cylinder by placing the constrictor ring around the base of the penis. This ring can be left in place for up to 30 minutes.

This technique requires a high level of manual dexterity and co-ordination. It is important that patients are adequately taught how to use their device, supplemented with written information. Most devices are now sold with an instructive video and, to maximise success rates, many manufacturers are offering educational support (teaching programmes) directly to patients if requested by the HCP. The success rate, that is an erection suitable for penetrative intercourse, appears to be very high if a robust vacuum device is used and sufficient training is provided. In some clinical studies, this success rate is as high as 90%. However, the quality of the erection is variable and unsatisfactory for some patients and their partners, and questionnaires have revealed a lower satisfaction rate (50%) compared with other treatment modalities.

Side-effects

These are listed in Table 9.1. Overall these are relatively minor and the drop-out rate is more related to the technique itself or quality of erection rather than the side-effect profile.

61

Table 9.1   Complications with the use of vacuum devices

Penile bruising
Ejaculation failure
Discoloration of the penis and the feeling of 'coldness'
Discomfort upon inducing a vacuum or application of the constriction band
Loss of acute angle of erection distal to constriction band

Surgery

The majority of cases of ED do not require surgical intervention. There are a few specific indications, however, in suitably screened patients.

Primary penile abnormalities

Primary penile abnormalities contributing to ED should be assessed by a urologist. These may include inherited conditions such as epispadias, curvatures or a micropenis. The most commonly encountered abnormality, however, is Peyronie's disease.

Peyronie's disease

Peyronie's disease occurs in up to 1% of the male population in middle age. It is characterised by fibrotic plaque formation within the penile shaft which is usually very evident on palpation of the penis during

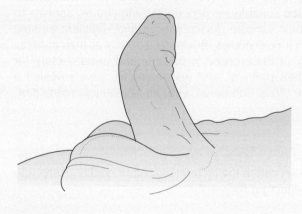

Figure 9.2
Peyronie's disease.
Typical angle on
erection.

examination. The aetiology of the condition is obscure but there is a familial tendency and there is an association with the presence of certain gene sequences. Trauma is also thought to feature in its development, leading to an inflammatory response and ultimately fibrosis. Clinical consequences also include penile pain and the development of angulation of the penis (see Figure 9.2).

Minor cases of Peyronie's disease may require no treatment or may respond to intracavernosal PGE1, thereby precluding the need for surgery. In some cases, surgery is required and can incorporate a range of techniques. In the Nesbit procedure, an ellipse of penile tissue (the tunica) is removed from the side opposite the most pronounced bend of the penile shaft and the remaining tissue edges rejoined. This removes the bend and in many patients may help to restore adequate tumescence. However, the patients need to be counselled appropriately since this technique inevitably shortens the penile length. Other procedures employed include plaque excision or incision coupled with grafting, whilst some patients may benefit from the insertion of a penile prosthesis.

Penile vascular surgery

These are highly specialised techniques carried out in a few urological centres. Success rates for revascularisation surgery depend upon the appropriateness of patient selection and experience of the surgeon and vary between 40 and 80%. Whilst it may be possible to improve penile blood flow, this does not necessarily imply reversibility of ED, in particular when there are associated abnormalities of penile smooth muscle relaxation. Diffuse atherosclerotic disease is less amenable to surgery compared with patients who have discrete arterial narrowings, the latter most commonly observed after pelvic trauma. These microsurgical techniques require the rerouting of a significant feeding blood vessel, most commonly the inferior epigastric artery which is anastamosed to vessels at the base of the penis.

The possibility of venous leakage and its diagnosis is discussed in Chapter 4. Venous surgery usually involves a combination of ligation and excision of offending veins. Success rates may be poor, resulting in the need for additional conventional treatment options reflecting the common finding of associated abnormalities of penile smooth muscle tone.

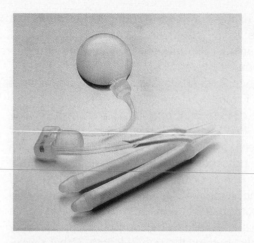

Figure 9.3   A penile prosthesis.

Penile prostheses

Penile prostheses (see Figure 9.3) are occasionally used for patients who fail to respond to other less invasive treatment. Alternatively, they may be used therapeutically in specific conditions such as patients with Peyronie's disease. Prostheses are inserted as a pair and generally made of a silicone rubber. There are three main types:

- *Malleable prostheses* are the cheapest and associated with the lowest failure rates. They contain silver wires within the silicone rubber which allow the semi-rigid penis to be bent into the most appropriate position.
- *Inflatable* and *mechanical* prostheses incorporate a mechanism which facilitates the ability to induce a flaccid or erect state, thereby eliminating the need for a semi-permanent erection. Given the more complex design of these devices, the mechanical failure rate is higher than that of malleable prostheses. In appropriately chosen

Table 9.2   Complications with the use of penile prostheses

Complications associated with the use of a general anaesthetic
Local complications (inadequate placement of the prosthesis, pain or infection)
Erosion of prosthesis in to local structures or externally
Mechanical failure of the prosthesis

patients, the success and satisfaction rates are high (60–90%). The side-effects associated with insertion of penile prostheses are shown in Table 9.2 but are rare, developing in less than 5% of patients and a similar percentage require further revision or replacement.

Key points

- Psychosexual counselling can be a useful first-line or additional approach in selected cases of ED.
- The most common treatment approach employs behavioural therapy, although cognitive therapy and psychoanalytical therapy may also be used.
- Vacuum devices offer a cost-effective and successful alternative to men in stable relationships but require adequate teaching and manual dexterity.
- Penile surgery is rarely required but may be useful for selected patients with penile abnormalities such as Peyronie's disease or vascular abnormalities.
- Penile prostheses are usually only inserted in patients requiring treatment for ED who have not been successful with less invasive approaches.

References and further reading

Cumming J, Pryor JP. (1991) Treatment of organic impotence. *British Journal of Urology* **67**, 640–3.

Masters WH, Johnson VE. (1970) *Human Sexual Inadequacy.* London: Churchill.

McLaren RH, Barrett DM. (1992) Patient and partner satisfaction with the AMS 700 penile prosthesis. *Journal of Urology* **147**, 62–7.

Montorsi F, Guazzoni G, Bergamaschi F, Rigatti P. (1993) Patient-partner satisfaction with semirigid penile prosthesis for Peyronie's disease. A 5-year follow-up study. *Journal of Urology* **150**(6), 1819–24.

Vrijhof HJEJ, Delaere KPJ. (1994) Vacuum construction devices in erectile dysfunction: acceptance and effectiveness in patients with impotence of organic or mixed aetiology. *British Journal of Urology* **74**, 102–5.

10 SPECIAL CONSIDERATIONS

Diabetes mellitus

Diabetes mellitus is the most common cause of ED, accounting for up to 40% of cases. Moreover, many of these patients (one in eight) may have previously undetected diabetes, justifying screening for this condition. At all ages, the presence of ED is greater in the diabetic compared with non-diabetic male (see Figure 10.1). Clinical factors most likely to be associated with its development include advancing age, treatment with insulin or oral hypoglycaemic agents, symptomatic autonomic or peripheral neuropathy or retinopathy.

Pathophysiology

This is complex and usually multifactorial. The common causes are shown in Table 10.1. Neurological factors have been implicated in 80% of ED cases in diabetic men. These abnormalities are almost exclusively

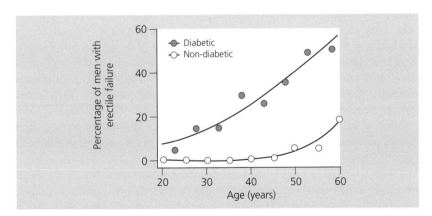

Figure 10.1   The prevalence of ED in patients with diabetes. Adapted with permission from Williams G, Pickup J. (2004) *Slide Atlas of Diabetes*. Oxford: Blackwell Science.

Table 10.1 Factors that may be, in particular, associated with the development of ED in diabetic men

Neural factors (predominatly, changes within the parasympathetic nervous system)
Vascular factors (atherosclerosis and endothelial dysfunction)
Functional and structural changes within the corpus cavernosum
Endocrine factors
Iatrogenic factors (drug use)
Psychological factors and psychiatric disorders
Infections (balanitis)

confined to the parasympathetic nervous system. The vascular supply to the penis may be affected by a generalised atherosclerotic process. More recently it has been identified that endothelial dysfunction may be responsible for inadequate blood flow. This impaired vascular reactivity is evident before the development of visible atherosclerotic plaques and can substantively reduce the penile blood supply when aroused, due to insufficient arterial dilation. The majority of diabetic men with ED have been shown to have some element of impaired blood flow.

Most interest has focused upon the smooth muscle abnormalities identified in diabetic men with ED. Increased fibrosis of the penile arteries, nerve fibres and corpus cavernosum is common, thereby attenuating typical penile vasodilation and smooth muscle relaxation. In addition, a number of changes in the availability or action of biochemical mediators that are involved in facilitating smooth muscle relaxation or constriction have been recognised. Reduced nitric oxide mediated smooth muscle relaxation has been observed as have prostanoid, vasoactive polypeptide (VIP) and adenosine triphosphate (ATP) mediated relaxation. Conversely, there may be alterations in noradrenaline, prostanoid and endothelin 1 mediated constriction that inhibit an erectile response.

Diabetic patients represent a population that is most likely to be on multiple drugs that may cause ED. There are several common culprits used in the treatment of diabetes or its complications (see Table 10.2). A more comprehensive list is found in Chapter 3. Thyroid disorders, associated with the development of ED, are more frequently observed in diabetic patients, although hypogonadism or hyperprolactinaemia is

Table 10.2   Drugs commonly prescribed in diabetic men that may cause ED

Cardiovascular protective drugs
   Thiazide diuretics and spironolactone
   Beta-blockers
   Angiotensin-converting enzyme inhibitors
   Calcium channel blockers and other antihypertensive agents
   Digoxin
Drugs for symptomatic relief of painful peripheral neuritis
   Tricyclic antidepressant agents
   Carbamazepine
   Gabapentin
   Non-steroidal anti-inflammatory agents
Lipid-lowering agents
   HMG CoA reductase inhibitors (statin therapy)
   Fibrates

no more common. Hyperglycaemia results in an increased incidence of balanitis in diabetes. Primary psychological disorders are a rare cause of ED in diabetes, although mixed organic and psychological factors are common. Structural changes in the penis, for example Peyronie's disease or venous leaks, have the same incidence in the diabetic and non-diabetic population.

Management

As usual, the history, examination and investigations should be conducted as outlined in Chapter 4. In clinical practice the management strategy is in most cases no different from that of the non-diabetic male with ED. However, there are a few practical considerations worthy of mention.

Glycaemic control in diabetes

Although poor glycaemic control is associated with a greater risk of ED, there is no evidence that improving glucose levels will reverse the condition. This is consistent with the general non-reversible nature of other diabetic complications such as neuropathy and nephropathy. In some situations, a transient precipituous deterioration in glycaemic control may be associated with the temporary development of ED, which may improve once optimal glucose control is re-established.

The presence of diabetic vascular complications

Diabetes is associated with a two- to fourfold increase in cardiovascular disease. Thus, its presence and severity of disease as well as risk of development needs to be assessed carefully before embarking upon treatment (see Chapters 4 and 5). In patients with significant retinopathy, the use of treatment such as vacuum devices may be restricted depending upon the degree of visual impairment. Very rarely, this may also apply to patients who have neuropathy involving the hands or advanced Dupuytren's contractures.

Effectiveness of treatment

As with non-diabetic patients with ED, oral therapy with PDE5 inhibitors is usually the first line of treatment. Their effectiveness is reduced by the presence of diabetes, but this should not preclude their use since at least three out of five patients respond. Overall the effectiveness of all three PDE5 inhibitors (sildenafil, tadalafil and vardenafil) in diabetic patients appears to be equivalent in clinical practice and the choice of agent should lie with consideration of the most suitable pharmacokinetic profile and other factors associated with their use (see Chapter 7). Similarly, the effectiveness of sublingual apomorphine would also appear to be reduced in diabetic patients, although the efficacy of penile injection therapy is broadly equivalent in diabetic and non-diabetic men.

Hypogonadism and other endocrine disorders

Clinical suspicion of hypogonadism and the appropriate blood tests to undertake are described in Chapter 4. Low measures of free active testosterone are best made on 9–10 a.m. blood samples, given the diurnal variation in testosterone production, and should be confirmed on repeat sampling. In most cases the low testosterone concentration is associated with elevated LH concentration, indicating the primary problem lies with the production of testosterone *per se* by the testes (primary hypogonadism). Occasionally, a low testosterone concentration is associated with a low LH or an LH value within the normal range (which may be considered inappropriately low) indicating a failure within the pituitary or less commonly the hypothalamus (secondary hypogonadism, see Table 10.3).

Table 10.3 Classification of hypogonadism

Primary	Secondary
Viral orchitis	Pituitary tumours (or their treatment)
Trauma	Craniophayngiomas
Castration	Isolated gonadotrophin deficiency
Anorchia	Haemochromatosis
Undescended testes	Sarcoidosis
Androgen resistance syndromes	Hyperprolactinaemia
Klinefelter's syndrome	Kallman's syndrome
Myotonic dystrophy	
Renal failure	
Drugs	

Secondary hypogonadism requires further evaluation of the pituitary, usually with magnetic resonance imaging as well as visual field and acuity assessment if a structural lesion is identified. Other hormone assessment is undertaken to assess pituitary reserve, either involving random sampling or dynamic pituitary testing. These investigations are best supervised by an endocrinologist in collaboration with an ophthalmologist and neurosurgeon where appropriate. If a pituitary tumour is identified, particular note of the prolactin measure should be made. A prolactin-secreting adenoma usually responds to medical therapy with dopamine agonists such as cabergoline, bromocriptine or quinagolide, resulting in tumour shrinkage, normalisation of prolactin concentrations and restoration of a normal testosterone axis. Elevated prolactin concentrations may be seen also in pituitary stalk compression, renal failure, hypothyroidism and with drugs that promote prolactin release (for example metoclopramide).

Testosterone replacement

Testosterone replacement is available in several forms (see Table 10.4). Oral therapy is relatively ineffective given the short half-life of approximately 90 minutes. The most commonly used and cheapest preparation remains deep intramuscular depot injections, usually administered into the buttock at intervals of 2–3 weeks. Pain associated with the

71

Table 10.4 Methods of testosterone replacement

Oral
Buccal
Intramuscular
Transdermal (patches or gel)
Subcutaneous pellet implants

injections can be troublesome and the 'yo-yo' response curve corresponds with peak levels achieved a few days after injection followed by a trough prior to the next. This cyclical response can be overcome in part by altering the time interval between injections and titrating dosage. Topical testosterone is available in either patch form or gel. The former is associated with a high incidence of skin irritation compared with the latter. Both forms are relatively expensive but have the advantage in most cases of achieving satisfactory constant physiological replacement doses of circulating testosterone. Within the UK, a buccal preparation, requiring replacement every 12 hours, has recently been launched, although clinical experience with this form of testosterone replacement is currently limited. Finally, some patients find the proposition of subcutaneous pellets inserted within the abdominal cavity wall appealing since they only need to be replaced every 6 months. All preparations require monitoring, particularly with regard to prostatic disease, which is more common in the over 50 years age group, where it is advisory to undertake palpation of the prostate and measure a prostatic specific antigen (PSA) concentration on an annual basis.

It should be noted that there is no place for testosterone treatment in patients with a normal testosterone axis. Opinion remains divided as to the use of testosterone in a patient with a 'low normal' circulating testosterone level associated with a normal LH concentration. This pattern of blood tests is commonly associated with the ageing male but if ED is reported associated with a reduction in libido, an empirical trial of testosterone over a period of 2–3 months with careful assessment may be justified.

Conventional treatment of thyrotoxicosis or hypothyroidism usually results in spontaneous resolution of ED without any further specific treatment.

Iatrogenic causes – drug therapy

Chapter 3 lists the drugs that have been implicated in the development of ED. However, use of these drugs does not necessarily imply a causal relationship. In our own experience, only patients in whom there is a clear temporal relationship between the initiation of a causative drug and ED (usually less than 2 weeks) respond to cessation of the drug. Moreover, in many instances a balanced judgement has to be made as to whether withdrawing the potential offending drug is feasible in light of the reason to commence it and whether alternative drug preparations less likely to cause ED are available. In many patients in whom it may not be possible to stop implicated drug therapy, traditional management routes should be offered.

Patients who do not respond to available treatment regimens

With advances in our understanding of the pathophysiology of ED and its management, it is fortunate that most patients can be treated satisfactorily. Many patients may have tried different treatment modalities before suitable therapy is identified. In some patients this may have required a combination of approaches, for example, both oral drug therapy and psychosexual counselling, or a combination of surgery and penile injection therapy in patients with Peyronie's disease.

Expectations of a positive outcome by the patient are also high, supported by the media hype around the treatment of ED. Such high expectations should be encouraged, reinforcing the likelihood of success with treatment found to be highly effective in clinical trials. It is always disappointing, therefore, when faced with a minority of patients who have not responded or tolerated the treatment options previously described in this book. In these cases, careful consideration must be given to the impact of unsuccessful treatment on the patient and partner and their quality of life. Psychological support should be offered where appropriate to help them come to terms with their limitations. Although satisfactory tumescence may not be achieved, an active sex life, which does not necessarily involve vaginal penetration, should be discussed and encouraged.

Key points

- Diabetes mellitus is the most common cause of ED, accounting for 40% of cases.
- The aetiology of ED is complex and often multifactorial. The most common implicated factors include neurovascular abnormalities and changes in the structure of the penis and impairment of smooth muscle relaxation.
- Treatment of diabetic patients with ED is usually no different from that of the non-diabetic male, although responses to therapeutic options are reduced.
- Identification of hypogonadism, hyperprolactinaemia and thyroid disease is important in patients with ED since their treatment is often associated with restoration of tumescence without the need for specific ED-related treatment.
- Cessation of offending drug therapy implicated in the development of ED may be considered. A clear temporal relationship between ED and the onset of the drug needs to be identified and whether it is safe to stop the causative drug.
- In the minority of patients who do not respond or tolerate treatment for ED, sexual activity involving non-penetrative intercourse should be encouraged and psychological support be offered if appropriate.

Further reading

Alexander WD, Cummings MH. (1996) Erectile dysfunction and its treatment. In: Shaw KM (ed.), *Diabetic Complications*. Chichester: John Wiley & Sons.

Cummings MH. (2004) Erectile dysfunction in diabetes. In: DeFronzo RA, Ferrannini E, Keen H, Zimmet P. (eds), *International Textbook of Diabetes*, 3rd edn. Chichester: John Wiley & Sons.

Goldstein I, Young JM, Fischer J. (2001) Vardenafil, a new highly selective PDE-5 inhibitor, improves erectile function in patients with diabetes mellitus. *Diabetes* **50**(2), 114.

Heaton JP, Lording D, Liu SN, Litonjua AD. (2001) Intracavernosal alprostadil is effective for the treatment of erectile dysfunction in diabetic men. *International Journal of Impotence Research* **13**, 317–21.

McCulloch DK, Campbell IW, Wu FC, Prescott RJ, Clarke BF. (1980) The prevalence of diabetic impotence. *Diabetologia* **18**, 279–83.

McCulloch DK, Young RJ, Prescott RJ, Campbell IW, Clarke BF. (1984) The natural history of impotence in diabetic men. *Diabetologia* **26**, 437–40.

Rendell MS, Rajfer J, Wicker PA, Smith MD. (1999) Sildenafil for treatment of erectile dysfunction in men with diabetes: a randomised control trial. *Journal of the American Medical Association* **281**, 424–6.

Saenz de Tejada I, Anglin G, Knight JR, Emmick J. (2002) Effects of tadalafil on erectile dysfunction in men with diabetes. *Diabetes Care* **25**(12), 2159–64.

.

11 WHAT ADDITIONAL SUPPORT IS AVAILABLE FOR MYSELF AND MY PATIENTS?

For many patients with ED, misconceptions both of the patients and HCPs have restricted successful treatment of this condition. Undoubtedly the situation has changed, but the greater the availability of accurate information, the more informed the individual becomes in managing or being treated for ED. Conversely, this can occasionally be counterproductive through inappropriate claims in the media or incorrect information on unofficial websites.

In addition to information provided by local clinicians, there are a number of peer-reviewed medical journals that report clinical studies and reviews on ED in specialty journals as well as general medical journals. These include:

- Urology journals: examples include *Journal of Urology, European Journal of Urology,* and *British Journal of Urology International*
- Diabetes journals: examples include *Diabetes Care, Diabetic Medicine, Practical Diabetes International, Diabetologia* and *Diabetes in Primary Care*
- Psychosexual journals: examples include *International Journal of Impotence Research, Archives of Sexual Behaviour, Journal of Sexual Medicine* and *Sexual and Relationship Therapy.*

The world wide web gives access to these journals on line through medical search engines such as 'Medline', 'Embase' and 'PubMed'.

Most of the pharmaceutical companies involved in treating ED are able to provide the relevant research literature as well as informative patient leaflets. Some have set up non-promotional patient websites.

In addition, many patient organisations provide telephone advice or patient literature on the management of ED. Examples include:

- Sexual Dysfunction Association (formerly The Impotence Association), Windmill Place Business Centre, 2–4 Windmill Lane, Southall, Middlesex UB2 4NJ. Tel: 0870 7743571 (http://www.sda.uk.net/)

- Diabetes UK, Diabetes UK Central Office, 10 Parkway, London NW1 7AA. Tel: 020 7424 1000; Fax 020 7424 1001 (http://www.diabetes.org.uk/home.htm)
- Diabetes Wellness and Research Foundation, Office 101–102, Northney Marina, Hayling Island, Hampshire, PO11 0NH. Tel: 023 9263 7808; Fax: 023 9263 6137 (www.diabeteswellnessnet.org.uk).

In the 1960s ED was just as common as it is now, but rarely discussed or treated. As HCPs in the new millenium, we are now at the stage of ensuring that every patient with ED benefits from the availability of modern information technology and an array of effective treatment options.

INDEX

Note: page numbers in *italics* refer to figures and tables

adenosine triphosphate   68
α-1-adrenergic agent   55
α-adrenergic receptor agonists   8
alcohol-related damage   16
Alzheimer's disease   16
cyclic AMP   11, 52
amyloidosis   16
angina   26, 35
antihypertensive agents   18–19
anxiety   2, 27
aorto-iliac surgery   20
apomorphine   47–8, 70
arterial surgery, reconstructive   32
atherosclerosis   17, 68
autonomic nerve testing   32
autonomic neuropathy   16, 26, 28

balanitis   20, 27
  diabetes   69
behavioural therapies   60
bitemporal hemianopia   29
bladder
  carcinoma   20
  innervation   26
bromocriptine   71
bulbocavernosal reflex   28, 29

cabergoline   71
capillary perfusion   28
cardiovascular disease   3, 27
  diabetes   70
  management   36
cardiovascular examination   28
cardiovascular fitness   26, 35, *36*
cardiovascular reflexes   32
cardiovascular risk   *37*
carotid bruits   28
causes of ED   15–21
cavernosal arteries   28
cavernosography   32

central nervous system (CNS) diseases
  16
cerebrovascular disease   28
cognitive therapy   60
communication in relationships   60
coronary disease   25
corpus cavernosum
  biochemical determinants of smooth
    muscle tone   18
  hypoxic damage   54
counselling
  psychosexual   59–60
cyproterone   19
cystectomy, radical   20

D2 receptor agonists   8
D2 receptors   47
  side-effects   *47, 48*
dementia, non-vascular   16
demyelination   16
Department of Health guidance on
    treatment   38–9
depression   2
detumescence   10
diabetes mellitus   3, 17, 25, 67–70
  autonomic neuropathy   16, 26, 28
  glycaemic control   69
  management   36, 69–70
  pathophysiology   67–9
  PDE5 inhibitors   45
  penis structure   18
  screening   29–30
  treatment of ED   70
  vascular complications   70
  vascular disease   28–9
diabetic ketoacidosis   26
dialysis   21
dopamine   8
dopamine agonists   71
dopamine receptors   47

79

Doppler ultrasound of penis   31
drug history   26–7
drug-induced ED   18–20, 73
  diabetes   68–9
Dupuytren's contractures   70
dyslipidaemia   25

endocrine examination   28–9
endocrine factors   17
endothelial dysfunction   17, 68
epididymal cysts   28
epigastric artery, inferior   63
epilepsy   16
epispadias   62
erections, spontaneous   25
exercise   3

follicle-stimulating hormone (FSH)   30
free androgen index   30

genitalia   27–8
glans penis   27, 28
cyclic GMP   11, 52
gynaecomastia   26, 29

haemoglobin, glycated (HbA1c)   30
heart disease, ischaemic   28
hydrocoeles   28
5-hydroxytryptamine (5-HT)   8
hyperglycaemia   69
hyperlipidaemia   17
hyperprolactinaemia   17, 21, 29
  diabetes   68–9
  management   37
hypertension   17, 25
hypnotic agents   20
hypogonadism   17, 21, 26, 28, 29
  classification   71
  diabetes   68–9
  investigations   70
  management   37
  screening   30
  secondary   71
hypotension, postural   26
hypothalamus   7–8, 9, 70
  chemical messengers   8

hypothyroidism   29, 71
  treatment   72

iatrogenic factors   18–20
information sources   77–8
International Index of Erectile Function
  (IIEF)   24
intracavernosal injection testing   30
intracorporeal self-injection therapy
  (ICSIT)   51–5
  consent   54
  effectiveness   54
  injection site   53, 54
  mechanism of action   52
  side-effects   54–5
  teaching   52–3
  technique   52–4
intracranial pressure, raised   26

journals   77

libido   7, 8
  CNS diseases   16
  enhanced   9
  impedance   17
  loss   26
  reduced   26
luteinising hormone (LH)   30, 70

macrovascular disease   25, 28–9
malignancy   16
metabolic equivalent of task (MET)   35,
  36
metoclopramide   71
micropenis   62
microvascular disease   28–9
MUSE (Medicated Urethral System for
  Erection)   55–7
  application   56
  effectiveness   56–7
  side-effects   57
myocardial infarction   26, 35

National Institute for Clinical Excellence
  (NICE)   3
Nesbit procedure   63
neural factors   16

neurological disease   27
neurological examination   28
neurological factors   26
neuropathy
    diabetic patients   70
    see also autonomic neuropathy
neurovascular factors   21
nicorandil   36, 46
nitrate therapy   36, 46
nitric oxide   11, *12,* 68
    metabolism disturbance   18

orgasm, sympathetic nerve stimulation
    9–10

pain
    penis   20, 57
    testosterone injection   71–2
papaverine   30
    injectable   51, 53
papillary dilation   32
papilloedema   29
parasympathetic nervous system   17
parkinsonism   16
patient assessment
    drug history   26–7
    general observations   23
    history   23–7
    investigations   29–32
    medical history   25–6
    physical examination   27–9
    problem definition   23–4
    psychological effects   27
    speed of onset   25
penile arteries   9
    fibrosis   68
penile arteriography   32
penile carcinoma   18
penile erections   7–12
    multiple organ co-ordinated response
        7–9
    physiological mechanisms within penis
        9–10
penile injections see intracorporeal self-
    injection therapy
penile prostheses   63, 64–5
    side-effects   *64,* 65

penile shaft, fibrotic plaques   27, 62–3
penile strain gauge   31
penile vascular surgery   63
penis
    acquired conditions   18
    assessment   27, 28
    blood flow restriction   16–17
    blood supply   9
    congenital conditions   18
    curvature   62
    Doppler ultrasound   31
    innervation   26
    neurovascular supply interruption   18
    nocturnal rigidity   31
    pain   20, 57
    previous surgery   17
    primary abnormalities   38, 62–3
    revascularisation   63
    smooth muscle
        constriction   11, *12*
        dysfunction   21
    smooth muscle relaxation   10–11, *12*
        ICSIT   52
        primary disorders   17–18
        reduced in diabetes   68
    structure changes in diabetes   18
    trauma   18
    vascular supply in diabetes   68
    venous drainage abnormalities   17
    venous leakage   30, 32, 63
performance anxiety   2, 15, 35
peripheral pulses   28
peripheral vascular disease   28
Peyronie's disease   17, 18, 27, 62–3
pharmacological therapy, invasive   51–7
phentolamine   53
phenylephrine   55
phimosis   27
phosphodiesterase type 5 (PDE5)
    inhibitors   2, 43–7
    contraindications   36
    diabetic patients   70
    economics   3–4
    efficacy   45
    pharmacokinetic properties   44, *45*
    prescriptions   39
    side-effects   45–6

phosphodiesterase type 5 (PDE5)
inhibitors (*cont.*)
tolerability   45–6
use   46–7
phosphodiesterase type 6 (PDE6)   46
pituitary gland   *9, 70, 71*
tumour   71
pituitary stalk compression   71
priapism   51, 54–5
risk   54
primary care   2
drug budgets   4
management   23
specialist care interface   39–40
prolactin   9
elevation   71
measurement   30
pituitary tumour secretion   71
prostaglandin E1   11, *12*, 30
injectable   51, 53–4
intracavernosal   63
intraurethral pellets   55–6
prostanoids   68
prostate
carcinoma   20
examination   29
radiotherapy   26
prostate disease   26
prostatectomy   20, 26
prostate-specific antigen (PSA)   72
prostheses   63, 64–5
psychiatric disorders   38
psychoanalytical therapy   60
psychogenic ED   20
psychological disorders   38
psychological factors   20, 21
diabetes   69
speed of onset   25
psychosexual counselling   59–60

quinagolide   71

radiological testing, invasive   32
radiotherapy, prostate   26
radiotherapy-induced ED   20
rectal carcinoma   20
rectal resection   20

referral of patients   40
renal failure, chronic   21, 71
renal transplant   20
retinopathy, diabetic   70

secondary sexual characteristics
absence   29
loss   26
self-esteem   27
self-image   27
sensate focusing   60
sepsis   26
sex hormone binding globulin (SHBG)   30
sexual activity, exertion level   35, *36*
sexual dysfunction, discussion   1–2
sildenafil   *4*, 43
diabetic patients   70
pharmacokinetic properties   44, *45*
side effects   46
smoking   17, 25
smooth muscle
constriction   11, *12*
dysfunction   21
smooth muscle relaxation   10–11, *12*
ICSIT   52
primary disorders   17–18
reduced in diabetes   68
snap gauge   31
specialist centres   2, 23, 39–40
spinal cord compression   16
spinal cord disease   16
spironolactone   19
surgery   62–5
surgery-induced ED   20
sweat spot test   32
sweating, gustatory   26
sympathetic nerve stimulation   9–10
systemic vascular disease   25

tadalafil   43
diabetic patients   70
pharmacokinetic properties   44, *45*
side effects   46
temporal lobe epilepsy   16
testes   *9*
examination   27–8
small   29

testosterone 8–9
   action inhibition 19
   diurnal variation 70
   measurements 30
   release inhibition 20
   replacement 71–2
thyroid 17
   metabolism 9, 29
thyroid disease management *37*
thyroid disorders 26
   diabetes 68–9
thyroid hormone concentrations 30
thyrotoxicosis 29
   treatment 72
tranquillisers 20
transurethral therapy 55–7
   side-effects 57
trauma
   penile 18
   Peyronie's disease 63
   spinal cord 16
treatment
   barriers 1–2
   Department of Health guidance 38–9
   economic considerations 3–4
   oral 43–8
   patients not responding 73
   physical benefits 3
   psychological benefits 2–3
   psychosexual counselling 59–60
   surgery 62–5

see also pharmacological therapy,
   invasive; phosphodiesterase type 5
   (PDE5) inhibitors; vacuum devices

urethroplasty 20

vacuum devices 60–1, *62*
   diabetic patients 70
   side-effects 61, *62*
   use 61
Valsalva manoeuvre 28
vardenafil 43
   diabetic patients 70
   pharmacokinetic properties 44, *45*
   side effects 46
varicocoeles 28
vascular disease
   premature 17
   risk factors 25
vascular disorders 3, 25–6
vascular factors 16–17
vascular insufficiency 26
vasoactive intestinal peptide (VIP) 11,
   12, 68
venous drainage abnormalities 17
venous leakage 30, 32, 63
visual fields examination 29
vitamin B12 deficiency 16

warfarin 36
websites 77